The No Breakfast Plan ar

by

Edward Hooke

PREFACE.

This volume is a history, or a story, of an evolution in the professional care of the sick. It begins in inexperience and in a haze of medical superstition, and ends with a faith that Nature is the all in all in the cure of disease. The hygiene unfolded is both original and revolutionary: its practicality is of the largest, and its physiology beyond any possible question. The reader is assured in advance that every line of this volume has been written with conviction at white heat, that enforced food in sickness and the drug that corrodes are professional barbarisms unworthy of the times in which we live.

E. H. DEWEY.

MEADVILLE, PA., U. S. A., November, 1900.

CONTENTS.

THE NO-BREAKFAST PLAN.

I.

PAGE

Introduction--Army experiences in the Civil War--Early years in general practice--Difficulties encountered--Medicinal treatment found wanting as a means to superior professional success 13

II.

A case of typhoid fever that revolutionized the Author's faith and practice--A cure without drugs, without food--Resulting studies of Nature in disease--Illustrative cases--A crucial experience in a case of diphtheria in the Author's family 26

III.

A study of the brain from a new point of view--Some new physiology evolved illustrated by severe cases of acute disease 34

IV.

The error of enforced food in cases of severe injuries and diseases illustrated by several striking examples 42

V.

An apostrophe to physicians 56

VI.

The origin of the No-breakfast Plan--Personal experience of the Author as a dyspeptic--His first experience without a breakfast--Physiological questions considered--A new theory of the origin and development of disease and its cure--The spread of the No-breakfast Plan--Interesting cases 60

VII.

Digestive conditions--Taste relish--Hunger relish--The moral science involved in digestion as a new study--Cheer as a digestive power--Its contagiousness--The need of higher life in the home as a matter of better health--Cheer as a duty 81

VIII.

The No-breakfast Plan among farmers and other laborers--A series of voluntary letters to an eminent divine, and the writer put down as a crank--The origin of the Author's first book--How the eminent Rev. Dr. George N. Pentecost was secured to write the introduction--His no-breakfast experience--The publisher converts a prominent editor--The case of Rev. W. E. Rambo, a returned missionary--The publishers' missionary work among missionaries-- The utility of the morning fast--Its unquestionable physiology--Why the hardest labor is more easily performed and for more hours without a breakfast 85

IX.

The utility of slow eating and thorough mastication unusually illustrated by Mr. Horace Fletcher, the author--What should we eat?--The use of fruit from a physiological standpoint 105

X.

Landscape-gardening upon the human face--A pen-picture-- Unrecognized suicide--Absurdity of the use of drugs to cure diseases--A case of blood-letting--Mission of homoeopathy-- Predigested foods 110

THE FASTING-CURE.

XI.

The forty-two day fast of Mr. W. W. C. Cowen, of Warrensburg, Ill., and its successful end--Press account--The twenty-eight day fast of Mr. Milton Rathbun, of New York, and its successful end--Press account--A second fast of Mr. Milton Rathbun, of thirty-five days, in the interest of science, and its successful end--Press account--Adverse comments of Dr. George N. Shrady, an eminent New York physician 117

XII.

The remarkable fast of forty-five days of Miss Estella Kuenzel, of Philadelphia, resulting in a complete cure of a case of melancholia--Press accounts--A still more remarkable fast, of fifty days, of Mr. Leonard Thress, of Philadelphia, resulting in a complete cure of a bad case of general dropsy--Press accounts--General dropsy in a woman of seventy-six relieved by a fifteen-day fast, with the cure permanent--Rev. Dalrymple's fast of thirty-nine and one-half days without interruption of pastoral duties 136

XIII.

Insanity--A study from a new point of view--Its radical cure deemed probable in most cases by protracted fasts--Feeding the insane as practised in the hospitals sharply criticised--Some direct words to physicians in charge 157

XIV.

The evolution of obesity, and its easy relief by fasting-- Overweight prevented by a limitation of the daily food and without lessening any of the powers or energies--The evolution and prevention of apoplexy 177

XV.

Chronic alcoholism--The evolution of the drunkard--His complete, easy, rational cure by fasting--No case so grave as to be beyond cure by this means--Asthma; Its cure through dietary means--A railroad tragedy--The need of railroad men to save their brains from needless waste of energy in their stomachs--An illustrative case--Some of the Author's troubles from the ignorance of the people--The death of Mrs. Myers, of Philadelphia, on the thirty-fifth day of her fast--Adverse press accounts and comments--Adverse comments of Prof. H. C. Wood, M. D., L. L. D., on fasting and fasters 183

XVI.

A successful sixty-day fast under the Author's care--More about predigested foods--Bathing from a physiological standpoint--The error of drinking water without thirst--Some earnest words to the mothers of this land--What the No-breakfast Plan means for them and their children--Concluding words 199

I.

A hygiene that claims to be new and of the greatest practicality, and certainly revolutionary in its application, would seem to require something of its origin and development to excite the interest of the intelligent reader. Methods in health culture are about as numerous as the individuals who find some method necessary for the health: taking something, doing something for the health is the burden of lives almost innumerable. Very few people are so well that some improvement is not desirable.

The literature on what to eat and not to eat, what to do and not to do, on medicines that convert human stomachs into drug-stores, is simply boundless. If we believe all we read, we must consider the location we are in before we can safely draw the breath of life; we must not cool our parched throats without the certificate of the microscope. We must not eat without an ultimate analysis of each item of the bill of fare, as we would take an account of stock before ordering fresh goods; and this without ever knowing how much lime we need for the bones, iron for the blood, phosphorus for the brain, or nitrogen for the muscles. In short, there is death in the air we breathe, death in the food we eat, death in the water we drink, until, verily, we seem to walk our ways of life in the very valley and shadow of death, ever subject to the attack of hobgoblins of disease.

How many lives would go down in despair but for the miracles of cure promised in the public prints, even in our best journals and monthlies, we cannot know. It is the hope for better things that sustains our lives; suicide never occurs until all hope has departed. Even our medical journals are heavily padded with pages of new remedies whose use involves the most amazing credulity. Perhaps it is well, in the absence of a sound physiological hygiene, that the people who are sick and afflicted shall be buoyed up by fresh, printed promises. Perhaps it is also well for the physician to be able to go into the rooms of the sick inspired from the advertising pages of his favorite medical journals.

Are they not new stars of hope to both physician and the people? Why should we not hope when new remedies are multiplying in such infinite excess over newly discovered diseases? New diseases? What is there essentially new that can be treated with remedies, in the coated tongues, foul mouths, high temperature and pulse, pain, discomfort, and acute aversion to food, that is to be found in the rooms of the sick? Are there really specifics for these conditions?

The hygiene to be unfolded in these pages is so new, so revolutionary, that its first impress has never failed to excite every form of opposition known to language, and yet its practicality is so great that it is rarely questioned by those who fairly test it. It has not been found wanting in its physiology, nor has it failed to grow wherever it has found lodgement.

The origin and development of this new way in health culture seem to require something of professional autobiography, that it may be seen that it is a matter of evolution and not of chance, not a fad that has only its passing hour.

After receiving my medical degree from the University of Michigan, and serving a term as house physician to the U. S. Marine Hospital at Detroit, Michigan, I entered one of the large army hospitals at Chattanooga, Tenn., at the beginning of the Sherman campaign in Georgia, where I found a ward of eighty sick and wounded soldiers fresh from the battle of Resacea. My professional fitness for duties so grave and so large in extent was of a very questionable order, and I did not in the least overestimate it.

It had not escaped my notice, even before I began the study of medicine, that whether disease were coaxed with doses too small for mathematical estimate, or whether blown out with solid shot or blown up with shells, the percentage of recoveries seemed to be about the same regardless of the form of treatment.

I was reared in a large family in a country home, several miles from a physician, where all but the severest sicknesses were treated with herb-tea dosage, and this was true of all other country homes. With all this in mind I had begun the study of medicine with a good deal less than the average faith in the utility of dosage, and it was not enlarged by my professor of materia medica.

I entered upon my serious duties as did good, rare, old Bunyan into his pulpit, with a feeling fairly oppressive that I was "the least of all the saints."

My materia medica was in my vest pocket; my small library in my head, with its contents in a very hazy condition. With a weak memory for details, and marked inability to possess truth except by the slow process of digestion and assimilation, my brain was more a machine-shop than a wareroom; hence capacity of retail dealing was of the smallest. I was not in the least conscious at this time that a large wareroom amply stored by virtue of a retentive memory was not the most needed as an equipment for all the practical affairs of life. I have ever found it necessary to dodge some memories, when there was lack of time to endure a hailstorm of details.

That I did not become a danger to the hapless sick and wounded only less than their diseases and wounds, was wholly due to my small materia medica, to utter lack of pride in knowledge that had not become a power with me, and to that lofty ambition for professional success which moved me to seize aid from no matter where or whom, as the drowning man a straw.

It was my great professional fortune that the medical staff of this hospital of more than a thousand cots was of a very high order of ability and experience, and that I entered at the beginning of a campaign in which for more than three months there was a fitful roar of artillery and rattle of musketry every day; hence a continuous influx to cots vacated by deaths or recoveries.

In all respects it was the best equipped hospital for professional experience of any that I knew anything about. There was one rigid rule that I believe was not carried out in any other hospital: post-mortems in all cases, numbering from one to a dozen daily, and all made with a thoroughness I have never seen in private practice.

The features of my hospital service that impressed me most were the post-mortem revelations and the diverse treatments for the same disease. I soon found that, no matter what the disease, every surgeon was a law to himself as to the quality, quantity, and times of his doses, with the mortality in the wards apparently about the same.

Post-mortem examinations often revealed chronic diseases whose existence could not have been suspected during life, and yet had made death inevitable.

Another advantage in army hospital practice was the stability of the position and the absence of the harassing anxiety of friends, thus affording the highest possibilities of the judgment and reason. And still another advantage was the high social relations existing between the medical officers, due to the absence of all causes for jealousy, neither the position nor salary depending on superior endowments or professional success.

I was aware that, in spite of my lack of experience and the presence of a most painful sense of general insufficiency, my sick and wounded were about as safe in my hands from professional harm, even from the first, as the patients of the most experienced medical officer in the hospital.

With high professional ideals, with no ability to make use of hazy conceptions or ideas, having no pride in knowledge that had not become my own, I began at once to reinforce myself from the experience and wisdom of my brother officers, whose advisory services were always readily and kindly rendered.

From the first and all through my military service my severely sick had the advantage of all the borrowed skill and experience I could command. As for surgical operations, they were all performed in the presence of most of the medical staff, some of whom were of great experience.

The surgery of the army hospitals of 1864 was of the highest character in skill and in careful attention to all the details involved, and the fatalities were generally due to the gravity of the wounds requiring operations and lack of constitutional power for recovery, rather than to the absence of the germ-killer. At that time the microbe was not a factor in the probabilities of life or death. In all else the care of the wounds could hardly be surpassed.

As for the medicinal treatment of my sick, it was unsatisfactory from first to last. After all the years since I cannot believe that, except for the relief of pain, any patient was made better by my dosage; and in all fatalities the post-mortem revealed the fact that the wisest dosage would have been without avail.

But in the study of the history of disease as revealed by symptoms my hospital experience was invaluable. I have since found that my greatest service at the beds of the sick is as an interpreter of symptoms rather than a vender of drugs. The friends of the sick read indications for good or bad with wonderful acuteness, as a rule; and I have rarely found myself mistaken in my ability to read the condition of patients in the faces of the friends, even before I enter the rooms of the sick.

As my experience enlarged so did my faith in Nature; and, since there was no similarity in the quality, sizes, and times of the doses for like diseases, my faith in mere remedies gradually declined.

After a year and a half of large opportunities to study the diseases of men in the early prime of life, in the care of the simple surgery of shot and shell, I left the army with such familiarity with grave diseases and death in various forms as to enable me ever after to retain complete self-possession in the presence of dying beds in private practice.

I began the general practice of medicine in Meadville in the autumn of 1866. Among the many physicians located in the city at that time were men of ability and large experience. There were those who administered with sublime faith doses too small for mathematical estimate; those who with equal faith administered boluses to the throat's capacity for deglutition; those who fully believed in whiskey as nourishment, that milk is liquid food, and who with tremendous faith and forceful hands administered both until human stomachs were reduced to barren wastes and death would result from starvation aggravated by disease.

Most of the cases of disease that fall to the care of the physician are trivial, self-limited, and rapidly recover under even the most crucifying dosages; Nature really winning the victories, the physician carrying off the honors.

This is so nearly true that it may be stated that, aside from the domain of surgery, professional success in the general sense depends upon the personal qualities and character of the physician rather than the achievements of the materia medica.

People have a confidence in the power of medicine to cure disease scarcely less than the dusky warrior has in the Indian medicine-lodge of the Western wilderness, and a confidence about as void of reason.

The physician goes into the rooms of the sick held to the severest accountability in the matter of dosage; and the larger his own faith in medicines the greater his task; and, if he is of my own, the so-called "old school," or Allopathic, the more dangerous he is to the curing efforts of Nature.

With the people the disease is simply an attack, and not the summing up of the results of violated laws going on perhaps from birth. With the people the symptoms are merely evidences of destruction, and not the visible efforts to restore the normal condition. Hence the failures to relieve always raise more or less questioning, among friends in painful concern, as to the ability of the physician to discharge his grave duties.

This unreasoning, unreasonable "blind faith" in remedial means is as strong in the most intelligent as in the most ignorant, and it has ever given me more trouble than the care of the sick. Another serious complication of the sick-room arises from near-by friends who are very certain that their own physicians are better fitted by far for the serious work of prescribing for the sick.

In addition to the serious work of attacking the symptoms of disease as so many foes to life, there is also a care as to what unbidden food shall go into unbidden stomachs, that the system shall be supported while life seems to be in the hands of its greatest enemy.

The universal conception of disease as a foe to life, and not as a rational process of cure; the boundless faith in remedies as means to resist the attack, revealed by symptoms, makes the professional care of the sick the gravest of all human occupations, and the most trying to both head and heart.

With all these taxing conditions confronting me, I opened an office in a field which seemed to be more than occupied by men of large experience.

With all my army experience I still had a hazy conception as to Nature in disease. That the vital forces needed the support of all the food the stomach of the sick could dispose of, was not a question of the remotest consideration. That medicine did in some way act to cure disease I could not fully question.

I was now to enter a service in which, from the care of infancy in its first breathings to old age in its last, every resource of the materia medica, of the reason, judgment, and of the soul itself, was to be called in in every grave case, and to be held to a responsibility measured by preposterous faith in medicines.

I entered upon my duties with a determination to win professional success by the most thorough attention to all the details of service upon the sick and their friends, and I confined my efforts almost wholly to acute cases. None of my professional colleagues were winning laurels by the treatment of chronic diseases, and not having faith in drugs for such I had my scruples about fees for failures that seemed inevitable.

And yet with the most painstaking service fortune would play with me at times in the most heartless manner. At one time four of my adult patients were awaiting burial within the radius of a half mile. As they were all physical wrecks, and died after short illnesses, there could be no question raised in any just sense as to the character of my services, but the fatalities were scored against me. Such fortune would be annihilating but for the fatalities inevitable with all practitioners.

For full ten years I visited the sick and dosed them according to the books, but with far less force of hands and faith than any of my brethren, and all were enjoined to take nourishment to keep up the strength for the combat with disease.

My doses were confined to only a few Sampsons of the materia medica, and these were administered with a watching for favorable results that could hardly be surpassed, and yet always with disappointment.

I was innocent enough to believe that a large practice could only be built up by the most painstaking and persistent effort; later on I found that a large practice was but little dependent upon the skill and learning displayed in the sick-room. One physician could immediately secure a large patronage because she was a woman; another, because he belonged to this or that nationality, or there was something in the personal outfit rather than in the professional that incited large hopes for the ailing.

In all my cases of acute sickness there was always a wasting of the body no matter how much they were fed; a like increase of general strength when a normal desire for food occurred no matter how little they were fed. I saw this with eyesight only; but I saw with insight that a large practice could be carried on by doctors too ignorant to know that there was an alphabet in medical science.

I was not then so fully aware of the depths of ignorance among the people as to what cures disease, did not know that faith in doses was so large, as child-like even with the most cultured as with the ignorant. I was not so well aware, as I became later, that the physician himself must have such energy of faith in the materia medica as to reveal it in every line of his countenance when in the rooms of the sick.

As the years went on, my faith in remedies did not increase; but I had to dose to meet the superstitious needs of the people. My practice, though far short of what it seemed to merit from the pains bestowed upon it, was large enough for all the needs of profitable study had I been in a condition for thought and reflection. It was not to my encouragement that there were those doing a far larger business with doses simply crucifying, and because crucifying, a far larger attendance was the direct result.

I now see, as I did not then so clearly, that Nature's victories are often won against the desperate odds of treatments that are simply barbarous; and yet Nature is so powerful, so persistent in the attempts to right all her wrongs, that she wins the victory in the great majority of cases no matter how severely she may be taxed with means that hinder. The great majority of the severely sick of a hundred years ago recovered in spite of the bloody lancet and treatments that are the barbarism of to-day.

II.

I was called one day to one of the families of the poorest of the poor, where I found a sick case that for once in my life set me to thinking. The patient was a sallow, overgrown girl in early maturity, with a history of several months of digestive and other troubles. I found a very sick patient, so sick that for a period of three weeks not even one drink of water was retained, not one dose of medicine, and it was not until several more days that water could be borne. When finally water could be retained my patient seemed brighter in mind, the complexion was clearer, and she seemed actually stronger. As for the tongue, which at first was heavily coated, the improvement was striking; while the breath, utterly foul at first, was strikingly less offensive. In every way the patient was very much better.

I was so surprised at this that I determined at once to let the good work go on on Nature's own terms, and so it did until about the thirty-fifth day, when there was a call, not for the undertaker, but for food, a call that marked the close of the disease. The pulse and temperature had become normal, and there was a tongue as clean as the tongue of a nursing infant.

Up to this time this was the most severely sick case I ever had that recovered, and yet with not apparently more wasting of the body than with other cases of as protracted sickness in which more or less food was given and retained. And all this with only water for thirst until hunger came and a complete cure!

Such ignoring of medical faith and practice, of the accumulated wisdom and experience of all medical history, I had never seen before. Had the patient been able to take both food and medicine, and I had prohibited, and by chance death had occurred, I would have been held guilty of actually putting the patient to death--death from starvation. Feed, feed the sick whether or not, say all the doctors, say all the books, to support strength or to keep life in the body, and yet Nature was absurd enough to ignore all human practice evolved from experience, and in her own way to support vital power while curing the disease.

I could recall a great many cases in which because of intense aversion to food patients had been sick for many days, and even weeks, with not enough nourishment taken to account for the support of vital power; but the fact did not raise a question with me.

The effect of this case upon my mind was so profound that I began to apply the same methods in Nature to other patients, and with the same general results. The body, of course, would waste during the time of sickness; but so did the bodies of sick that were fed. As for medicines, they were utterly ignored except where pain was to be relieved, though unmedicated doses were alike a necessity with all. Not a single medicine was given except for pain, and occasionally in cases in which I had reason to think the entire digestive tract needed a general clearing of foul sewage. Thence on, that supreme work, the cure of disease, in my hands became the work of Nature only.

In a general practice I was able to carry out the non-feeding plan by permitting the various meat teas or the cereal broths, none of which can be taken by the severely sick in quantities to do harm. By withholding milk I was enabled to secure all the fasting Nature required, while satisfying the ever-anxious friends with tea and broth diversions.

This was a line of investigation that I felt ought to be of the deepest interest to every thinking, high-minded physician, to every intelligent layman; and very early the evidences of the utility of withholding food from the sick during the entire time of absence of desire for it, its absolute safety, were beyond any questioning.

I had no fatalities that were apparently in any way due to the enforced lack of food. In cases of chronic disease in which death was inevitable, such as cancer, consumption, etc., patients were permitted to take what they could with the least offence to the sense of relish. In every case of recovery there was a history of increasing general strength as the disease declined, of an actual increase of vital power without the support of food that had no more relish than the dose that crucified the nerves of taste.

In all America milk is the chief reliance to support vital power when no other food can be taken. Milk in one stage of normal digestion gets into the form of tough curds ready for the press, and curds should always be thoroughly masticated before swallowing.

Sir William Roberts, of England, in his exhaustive work on Digestion and Diet, asserts that milk-curds are not digested in the stomach during sickness, but are forced into the duodenum, where, he asserts, they are digested, but he gives no reason for his faith that there is power to digest in the duodenum where there is none in the stomach.

It was not difficult to make the mothers in the homes understand that taking milk by the drink was equivalent to swallowing green cheese-curds without due mastication.

With these hygienic conceptions and methods I continued to visit the sick as a mere witness of Nature's power in disease rather than as an investigator, yet without being able to understand the secret of the support of vital power without food. But whatever risk there might be, or how strong my faith when my patrons were the subjects of what might be called foolhardy experiments, there came a time when this faith was to have the severest of all tests.

An epidemic of diphtheria broke out among my nearest neighbors, and after four deaths in as many families within a stone's throw of my residence a son of mine aged three years was taken. I had never given him in all his life even a cross look, and whatever sin there was in making idols of children in this I was the worst of all sinners, and I did not quite believe, as some Christian folks would have me, that my happiness through him was not the very incense of gratitude to the great Author for the gift of such a treasure of the heart.

In my hour of trial two of my ablest and most experienced medical friends came to me. Quinine and iron in solution were their verdict--and the little throat was not copper-lined; and, in addition, all the strong whiskey possible to force into the stomach: all this would have required manacled wrists and the prying apart of set jaws. He had never received anything from me more violent than caresses, and this abomination of dosage was to be sent down a bleeding, ulcerated way, over raw surfaces that would writhe and quiver under the added torture. This would not be rational treatment for ulcerations on the body, and the loss of strength through resistance and structural injury to the throat had no promise of redemption except in the minds of my medical friends.

It happened that I left home without getting the prescription filled, and, not getting back as soon as expected, the anxious wife procured the medicines and succeeded in getting one dose into the stomach, and also in raising a nervous hurricane that took an hour to allay. She was then informed that such a dose would be cruel even to a horse. Thence on he took nothing into his stomach but the water that thirst compelled, and a little dosage with it to meet the mother's need; and so I stood beside the suffering idol of my heart, with the entire medical world against me--strong enough, only rejoicing in my strength to defend him against the barbarism of authorized treatment. My only comfort was that in his time of supreme need I could give him supreme kindness, and if death must come there would not be the additional laceration of avoidable cruelty inflicted; and Nature, with every possible aid that could add comfort to the suffering body, won the victory.

Since then the medical world has advanced to antitoxin as a specific, leaving me nearly alone to plodding ways that are by sight and not by faith. That the treatment of my sick son in the absence of the only supposed specific was in advance of my time, the medical world cannot now question.

As the months and years went on, it so happened that all my fatalities were of a character as not to involve in the least suggestions of starvation, while the recoveries were a series of demonstrations as clear as anything in mathematics, of evolving strength of all the muscles, of all the senses and faculties, as the disease declined. No physician whose practice has been extensive has failed to have had cases in which the same changes occurred, and in which the amount of food taken did not explain this general increase of strength.

Believing I had made a most important discovery in physiology, one that would revolutionize the dietetic treatment of the sick, if not ultimately abolish it, my visits to the sick became of unsurpassed interest, I watched every possible change as an unfolding of new life, seeing the physical changes only as I would see the swelling buds evolve into the leaves or flowers, reading the soul- and mind-changes in the more radiant lines of expression.

I saw all these things with the naked eye, and more and more marvelled at the bulk of our materia medicas, the size of our drug-stores, and the space given to healing powers in all public and medical prints.

For years I saw my patients grow into the strength of health without the slightest clue to the mystery, until I chanced to open a new edition of Yeo's Physiology at the page where I found this table of the estimated losses that occur in death after starvation:

Fat 97 per cent. Muscle 30 " Liver 56 " Spleen 63 " Blood 17 " Nerve-centres 0

And light came as if the sun had suddenly appeared in the zenith at midnight. Instantly I saw in human bodies a vast reserve of predigested food, with the brain in possession of power so to absorb as to maintain structural integrity in the absence of food or power to digest it. This eliminated the brain entirely as an organ that needs to be fed or that can be fed from light-diet kitchens in times of acute sickness. Only in this self-feeding power of the brain is found the explanation of its functional clearness where bodies have become skeletons.

I could now go into the rooms of the sick with a formula that explained all the mysteries of the maintenance and support of vital power and cure of disease, and that was of practical avail. I now knew that there could be no death from starvation until the body was reduced to the skeleton condition; that therefore for structural integrity, for functional clearness, the brain has no need of food when disease has abolished the desire for it. Is there any other way to explain the power to make wills with whispering lips in the very hour of death, even in the last moments of life, that the law recognizes as valid?

I could now know that to die of starvation is a matter not of days, but of weeks and months; certainly a period far beyond the average time of recovery from acute disease.

III.

There fell to my care a very much worn-out mother, who took to her bed with an attack of inflammatory rheumatism, with the joints so involved as to require the handling of a trained nurse. The agony was such that the hypodermic needle was required to make existence endurable, and it was used with the idea that the brain would be less injured by the remedy than by the agony with its inevitable loss of sleep.

I know of no disease in which treatment has been more savage than in this. The remedies in common use at that time were mainly new and of supposed specific powers; but they were so violent, and proved to be so futile, that they have all been given up since by the majority of the profession.

As the days went on the disease declined in spite of the enforced comfort through the needle; there were easier movements, a clearing of the skin from sallow to a tint of redness, and finally, after a month, the armchair could be used for a change.

On the morning of the forty-sixth day there was revealed in the face the perfect color of health, and happiness marked every line of the expression. There was ability to walk through several rooms of her home. But it was not until the afternoon that the first food was desired and taken, and never before was plain bread and butter, the supreme objects of desire, so relished. In the following few months there was an actual gain of forty pounds.

My next marked case is a wonderful illustration of the self-feeding power of the brain to meet an emergency, and a revelation, also, of the possible limitations of the starvation period. This was the case of a frail, spare boy of four years, whose stomach was so disorganized by a drink of solution of caustic potash that not even a swallow of water could be retained. He died on the seventy-fifth day of his fast, with the mind clear to the last hour, and with apparently nothing of the body left but bones, ligaments, and a thin skin; and yet the brain had lost neither weight nor functional clearness.

In another city a similar accident happened to a child of about the same age, in whom it took three months for the brain to exhaust entirely the available body-food.

I will now enter upon a study of the brain and its powers along these lines, to be enlivened by illustrative evidence. What reason and physiology had I with me that I should use methods in the sick-room wherein the entire medical world was against me, and with severest condemnation?

The head is the power-house of the human plant, with the brain the dynamo as the source of every possible human energy. We think, love, hate, admire, labor with our hands, taste, hear, smell, see, and feel through the brain. Broken bones and wounds heal, diseases are cured through energy evolved in the brain or the brain system as a whole. The other so-called vital organs and the muscles are only as so many machines that are run by the brain power, with the stomach an exceedingly important machine. That powers so rare do not originate in the bones, ligaments, muscles, or fats, does not need argument; that when the nerve-trunks that supply the arm or leg are severed power of movement and feeling is lost, is known to all; and equally would the power of the stomach be abolished were the nerve-trunks cut off. In a general way, then, it may be stated that the strength of the body is directly as the strength of the brain.

With this physiology, who in or out of the medical profession can fail to see clearly that the digestion of even an atom of food is a tax upon the strength of the brain for whatever of power needed by the stomach, the machine, for this purpose? Unless it can be proved that the stomach has powers not derived from the brain system, this will have to be admitted.

How is the strength kept up in the light of this physiology? The universal belief is that it is kept up by the daily food. In proportion to the prostration of sickness, so are physicians anxious to conserve the energies by working the stomach to the limit of its powers.

The impression that there must be something digested to support the vitality of the system is a belief, a conviction that has always been too self-evident to suggest a doubt.

If the well need food to keep up the strength, the sick need it all the more; this is the logic that has been displayed upon this question. Let us keep it clear in mind that, if the nerves going to the stomach are severed, paralysis will result as in the case of the arm, in order more definitely to conceive the stomach as a machine that requires power to run it even to a tiringout degree. This is strikingly illustrated by the exhausted feeling that invites the after-dinner nap for rest, which, however, does not rest overfilled stomachs, overfilled brains. The brain gets no rest while getting rid of food-masses with more of decomposition than of digestion.

If food really has power to keep up the strength, there should not be so much strength lost by the general activities--indeed, it would seem that fatigue should be impossible. But the fact remains that from the first wink in the morning to the last at night there is a gradual decline of strength no matter how much food is taken, nor how ample the powers of digestion; and that there comes a time with all when they must go to bed, and not to the dining-room, to recover lost strength. The loss of a night of sleep is never made up by any kind of care in eating on the following day, and none are so stupid as not to know that rest is the only means to recover from the exhaustion of excessive physical activity.

The brain is not only a self-feeding organ when necessary, but it is also a self-charging dynamo, regaining its exhausted energies entirely through rest and sleep. There is no movement so light, no thought or motion so trivial, that it does not cost brain power in its action--and this is true of even the slightest exercise of energy evolved in digestion.

Why, then, do we eat?

For two reasons, or perhaps three: we eat because we are hungry. We rarely fail to eat excessively to satisfy the sense of relish after the normal hunger sense has been dissipated; we may eat to satisfy relish as we eat ice cream, fruits, and the enticing extras that beguile us to put more food into the stomach after it is already overfilled for its working capacity. But our actual need of food, the best reason for taking it, is to make up for the wastes from the general activities; and this is a process in the order of Nature that actually tires the entire brain system, or, in the common phrase, the whole body, unless the stomach has powers not derived from the brain system.

Now as we need not, cannot feed the brain in time of sickness, what can we feed? In all diseases in which there are a high pulse and temperature, pain or discomfort, aversion to food, a foul, dry mouth and tongue, thirst, etc., wasting of the body goes on, no matter what the feeding, until a clean, moist tongue and mouth and hunger mark the close of the disease, when food can be taken with relish and digested. This makes it clearly evident that we cannot save the muscles and fat by feeding under these adverse conditions.

Another very important, unquestioned fact is that disease in proportion to its severity means a loss of digestive conditions and of digestive power.

Cheer is to digestion what the breeze is to the fire. It may well be conceived that there are electric nerve wires extending from the depths of the soul itself to each individual gland of the stomach, with the highest cheer or ecstacy to stimulate the highest functional activity, or the shock of bad news to paralyze. From cheer to despair, from the slightest sense of discomfort to the agony of lacerated nerves, digestive power goes down. Affected thus, digestive power wanes or increases, goes down or up, as mercury in a barometer from weather conditions.

Digestive conditions in their maximum are revealed in the school-yard during recess, when Nature seems busy recovering lost time.

How compares the ramble of a June morning, with the blue and sunshine all above, the matchless green of the trees, and all the air fragrant with the perfume of flowers and alive with music from the winged singer, in digestive conditions, with those in the rooms of the sick, where there is only distress felt in the body and seen in the faces of the friends?

In time of health, if we eat when we are not hungry, or when very tired, or in any mental worriment, we find that we suffer a loss of vital power, of both physical and mental energy. How, then, can food be a support to vital power when the brain is more gravely depressed by disease? Yet from the morning of medical history the question of how vital power is supported in time of sickness has never been considered, because there has never been any doubt as to the support coming from food. I assume this to be a fact, since all works on the practice of medicine of to-day enjoin the need to feed the sick to sustain their depressed energies--all this without a question as to whether there is not a possibility of adding indigestion to disease when food is enforced against Nature's fiat.

Since vital power is centred in the brain, do we need to feed, can we feed, for other than brain reasons? This physiology admitted, there is no other conclusion possible than that feeding the sick is a tax on vital power when we need all that power to cure disease.

With all this physiology behind me, for more than a score of years I have been going into the rooms of the sick to see the evolutions of health from disease, as I see the evolutions from the dead wastes of March to the affluence of June, and from the first I had the exceeding advantage of being able to study the natural history of disease, a history in which none of the symptoms were aggravated by digestive disturbances.

As there was no wasting of vital power in the hopeless effort to save the body from wasting, I had a clear right to presume that my patients recovered more rapidly and with less suffering. With no perplexing study over what foods and what medicines to give, I could devote my entire attention to the study of symptoms as evidences of progress toward recovery or death; and in addition to all this there was the great satisfaction of being strictly in line with Nature as to when and what to eat.

As to the danger of death from mere starvation, the following remarkable case reveals how remote it is in the ordinary history of acute diseases. The late Rev. Dr. Merchant, of Meadville, Pa., a short time before his death, which occurred some months ago, informed me that a brother entered the army during the War of the Rebellion with a weight of one hundred and fifty-nine pounds. He was sent home so wasted from ulceration of stomach and bowels that he actually spanned his thigh with thumb and finger. He lived ten days only, to astonish all by the clearness of his mind even on the last day of his life, when he could think on abstruse questions as he had never been known to do in health. At death his body weighed only sixty pounds.

It was Dr. Merchant's opinion, from a history of the case, that no food was digested during the last four months of his life; but it is my opinion that it took a much longer time than this for the brain to absorb more than ninety pounds of the body. That life was shortened by the more rapid loss of the tissues from the disease is to be taken into account in estimating time in starvation.

IV.

Feeding the sick! Who that rule in kitchens and feed the well do not realize with weariness of brain the demands of the stomach that at each meal there shall be some change in the bill of fare?

The chief reliance of physicians for the maintenance of strength while sick bodies are being cured is milk. As a food, milk was mainly destined for the calf, and not for man--certainly not after the coming of the molars. It is not a food that will start the saliva in case of hunger, as the odors from the frying-pan or from roasting fowl, yet because it plays such an important part as a complete food for some months in the life of the calf, and because it can be taken without especial aversion when the odors of the cooking-stove are an offence to the nostrils; it is given by the hour, day after day, and in some cases week after week; and there are physicians by the thousands who reinforce this inflexible bill of fare by the strongest alcoholics, whiskey being generally selected.

In this connection I shall say of alcoholics that they contain not an atom that can be converted into living atoms; they congest and irritate the stomach, and hence lessen digestive power; and benumb all the brain powers and faculties.

As a daily ration without change, this combination, strictly adhered to, would prostrate the energies of a giant, and he would find himself mustered out of all active service in less time than the hapless sick are often compelled to endure such feeding. Does Nature so conveniently reverse herself to meet an emergency that the sick can be built up and sustained by such feeding as would debilitate the well?

In the city where I live the physicians average well in learning, ability, character, and experience. Among them are the extremists in dosage: those with a hundred remedies for a hundred symptoms; others with such boluses as would writhe the face of an ox. There are some with extraordinary force of command in the rooms of the sick, who believe that whiskey is nourishing and that milk is liquid food; that doses go into human stomachs to travel the rounds of the circulation, and finally drop off at the right place for either patchwork or original work.

Whatever there is in drugs to cure disease, whatever in milk and the strongest alcoholics to sustain the strength, every protracted case has been made to reveal in their forceful hands. I have no reason to believe they exceeded authorized treatments. I have no reason to doubt that in all countries, in all lands, where there are educated physicians, the same appliances are in common use, appliances that will make the next short step from the lancet and bolus of a darker age the estimate of the time to come.

The treatments of the sick are always changing, while the process of cure remains the same. Only in the case of broken bones are we compelled to let Nature do all the curing, while we may take pride in some progress in the mechanical appliances.

As milk and stimulants are a common, authorized means to sustain the sick, and as they are poured into human stomachs with all the faith with which lancets were once forced into congested veins, their efficiency for good or evil must be studied by comparison.

Treatments must lessen both the severity and the duration of disease to be of permanent benefit. For a study by comparison, this opportunity came to me. There was a call to attend a case of typhoid fever in a young girl. In the same vicinity there had been under the care of one of my forceful brethren a woman in middle life, whose stomach was habitually rejecting all the milk and alcoholics poured into it, the doctor having a theory that good would result no matter how brief the time they were retained.

For a month my patient swallowed only the desired water and doses which did not corrode, a desire for food coming at the end of the month. The only day and night nurse was an overwrought mother, who got into bed with the same disease as soon as the daughter got out of it. There was another month of severer sickness, when without food and without the horror of dosage, as before, the call for food marked the close of the disease. My services ended here some days before the undertaker took charge of the doctor's case.

A girl in her later teens, with a mild, so-called malarial fever, fell into the same forceful care. There was a true history in this case of nearly two gallons of whiskey, and daily milk from the quart at first down to inability to take the least nourishment at last. Then there were more than a month of days when vital power sustained itself without the ways of violence, death occurring during the nineteenth week.

The ravenous brain had absorbed the lips to such thinness that the depressions between the teeth were clearly revealed. From the first dose to the last breath this was a case of dying, and the most persistent fight for life against immense odds I have ever become aware of in an acute case. In this case the stomach had become so seared by the alcoholic that digestion was impossible, as would have been the case in a body that was not sick.

Near this home there was a more delicate girl of about the same age taken with the same fever; but with mild dosage and no food--in Nature's care--

hunger came at the close of the fourth week.

Later on in the same family there was a case of la grippe, in which for several years there had been chronic, ulcerative bronchitis that bid defiance to blisters and inhalations, the various specifics of another forceful predecessor, who also was a believer in large doses and full rations of alcoholized milk.

The coughing was so persistent, so continuous, that only the hypodermic needle met the need. To prevent the tearing of a raw surface in the bronchial tubes by the cough was as necessary as to apply splints to a broken bone. There was no food for six weeks, and Nature made most of her opportunity, not only to cure the acute disease, but also the chronic disease, which for nearly ten years since has remained cured.

I was summoned to Asheville, N. C., to see a young man in the last stage of consumption. I found him nearly a skeleton, though he had been eating six times daily for several months by the decree of a really learned physician. The belchings from gas were loud and frequent; the sputa by actual measure was about six ounces during every twenty-four hours.

A fast was ordered, and on the third day a mass of undigested food was thrown up. As soon as the stomach and bowels became empty there was comfort all along the line, and the cough was so diminished, that less than an ounce of sputa was raised in twenty-four hours.

After a week of fasting there came a natural desire for food, and thence on he enjoyed without distress of stomach all he wished to take. Thence on he lived with only the least discomfort, and with whispering lips he dictated to me his will, conveying large property. He could look with meaning when the power to whisper was gone, and life ended as the going out of a candle.

For months his sufferings had nearly all been due to food masses in a state of decomposition. He saw clearly and mentioned often that his had been a case of starvation from overfeeding. Nature finally had to succumb because she was not also able to deal with a clearly avoidable disease, indigestion; but she kept up a brave fight until the body was nearly absorbed.

As soon as the stomach and bowels became empty the friends noticed that nervousness largely disappeared. His sleeps were much longer, because not broken by coughing as before; and as the brain was not taxed with food masses there was an accumulation of power that was clearly revealed in the cheer of expression and a calmness as if heavenly rest had come at last.

A few years ago an attorney in this city had to endure a course of fever to which was added all the known barbarism of the times. Under enforced food and stimulants his mind at last became so weak that the dosings were forced down his throat. There were many weeks of life at lowest ebb before the man of torture (the doctor) was compelled to discontinue his evil work, and there were then months, extending to years, during which there appeared a colorless ghost of his former self on the streets--and this in spite of a wood-chopper's daily eatings, which were far in excess of power to digest.

At last he was brought to his couch with a mild fever complicated with a variety of other ailings. Not one of his friends who knew him intimately expected his recovery, as it was believed by them that there were chronic conditions that were beyond cure, and this because there had been death in manner, movements, and looks for months. And yet he had been able to take a stomach to his office every morning for many weeks filled with pancakes, sausage, fried potatoes, etc., only to shiver before the stove between his stomach-fillings.

To this possibly hopeless case I was called, and from that time he was to suffer only from the disease. For nearly three weeks no food was called for; and yet power so increased that he became able to dress himself; and on the morning before hunger finally called for food he came down from his bedroom with a son on his back who weighed not less than seventy-five pounds. Thence on, life, color, mind, muscle, rapidly came until there was such regeneration as to reveal a new body and a new soul.

Some years before this event an only son was taken sick with a mild fever. A young physician and friend of the patient was called whose faith in drugs, milk, and whiskey was boundless. He was fresh from his university, and therefore Nature had no part, through experience at the sick-bed, in the cure of disease. For many weeks these remedies of torture were vigorously and persistently enforced. But the time came when Nature would bear no longer.

The father, a personal friend, came to see me simply to unburden himself, and as he was not able to give me the case I was unprofessional enough to advise that the attendance should go on, but that there should be a complete rest the physician should not know of. This was done, and in a few days there was a call for food, the first call in more than two months. Of course, there was a recovery, which was an exceeding victory for Nature against extraordinarily adverse conditions, but it required many months to restore the wrecked balance.

As I write this experience the following comes to me as a still stronger indictment against authorized medical method. A. B., when in the early maturity of his physical manhood, was stricken with a partial paralysis that sent him to his bed. It was simply the case of a wound of the brain requiring rest as the chief condition for cure. But milk, whiskey, and drugs were used with the greatest persistence, and after three months he became able to be about, no less feeble in mind than in body, and with teeth utterly ruined by the dosage. For fully five years he went about his home and along the streets as one in a dream. For ten years there was inability to attend to his ordinary business. Life came at last through the no-breakfast plan.

The most remarkable fight for life on the part of Nature against the adverse conditions of drugs, alcoholics, and milk I have ever known was in the following case: A spare woman, of perhaps forty years, came to her bed the victim of habitual bromidia and chloral, invited by severe headaches. The treatment of this case was as follows: whiskey every hour, milk every other hour; corrosive medication and powerful brain sedative every night, which would have paralyzed digestive energy for many days. There was not an hour during the twenty-four in which there was not dosing either to cure the disease or to sustain the system. The average quantity of whiskey was six ounces daily, and of milk nearly a quart. This treatment was borne for weeks, merging into months. There was no disease not caused by the treatments, and the battle went on until there was only the shadow of a woman left when Nature rebelled against further violence. A few days of peace were granted because hope had departed; but it took Nature more than a year to recover from the damage.

A man of iron and steel, in the early prime of life, was the victim of a severe injury. With the agony of lacerated nerves and the hypodermic needle to make the digestion of food impossible, milk and whiskey were poured into an unwilling stomach from the first, and both were used until neither could be retained; and then the lower bowel was extemporized into a stomach. For one hundred and forty-six days, from three to seven doses of morphine were put into the arm daily; and morphine dries both mouth and stomach and lessens all energies of the brain. The body itself was not sick; there was no hint of disease in it; yet there were drugs prescribed that cost dollars by the score, and there were alcoholics by the gallon. For months the pain, alcoholics, and morphine kept the mind in such a daze that there were only the imbecilic mutterings of a dreamer in trouble.

The only treatment indicated in this case was the best of surgery for the injury, and some easing doses for a short while at first, to relieve pain. No food would be desired or digested; so the fast would go on until there would be a natural hunger, which would only manifest itself when there would be marked relief from pain. The meals, thence on, would be so far apart that all would be keenly relished; and there could be no loss of weight when meals would be so taken.

It is not surprising when I say that a seared stomach and a brain converted into a whiskey pickle had no part in the digestion of milk: else why did the weight of one hundred and sixty pounds at the time of the accident fall to eighty-five at the time of hunger? And all this drugging and alcoholics for a man who was not really sick! and the bill of fare that was not changed during one hundred and sixty days! and the time lost, and the expense entailed, and the anxious, aching hearts that were nearest the bed of horrors--of horrors, torments clearly invited.

By way of contrast the following case is given. During vacation a lad of twelve years of one of my families took to his bed with appendicitis in severe form. A learned physician was called, and there were many days of morphine, with other medication and all the food that could be coaxed into an unwilling stomach. Enough morphine was given daily to paralyze digestive energy for at least two or three days in one in ordinary health. There was a month of this war against Nature, when the violence of the acute attack subsided and a partial victory was gained against great odds.

On my return I found him under heavy dosage for the recovery of strength and lost appetite. Colorless, an鎚ic, languid--he was barely able to walk. He was immediately put under my care, and therefore under a fast that ended in a few days in such hunger as had not been felt in several months; and color, cheer, energy, weight evolved in a month. But there was also a developing abscess deep in the groin, and the time came when a grave operation was necessary to save life. He was made ready for the surgeon's knife that cut its way down, down many inches to relieve walls ready to burst from the tension. The wound remained in the care of the surgeon, but the life in my care. Who deny that the an鐺thetic, the shock of the operation, and the subsequent pain will not abolish all power to digest as well as all the desire for food? Here was a patient waiting for Nature to rally, which she did on the third day in a call for food; and thence on one daily meal was keenly relished, and the wound was healed--a wound that was three inches long on the surface and six inches deep. On the fifteenth day the lad was able to be dressed and able to walk about his room, and with a freshness of color that was never observed in him before. What law of body was violated in the preliminary treatment intended to prepare Nature for the ordeal and to enable her to rally from it?

This fresh tragedy in one human life has become known to me while I write. A man, a giant, in his eighty-eighth year, lost his appetite, and was put to death by the following means: A pint of whiskey and from one to two quarts of milk daily to keep him nourished. Five months passed without any change in the bill of fare--five months of delirium, of imbecilic muttering before the last breath was drawn. These tragedies are common the world over. Do I cry against them with too loud a voice? Would that I had a voice of thunder!

I have given a few examples of the crucifixions of the sick and the afflicted, whereof I have many, and they are the real history of cases known, and are constantly occurring in every community.

The cure of disease and injury by fasting--the mode of Nature--made the greatest impression in families in which there was intelligence enough to comprehend it; but the victories of Nature were complicated by cases in which death was inevitable. With a feeling that I must give the new hygiene to the world in printed form, I did not enlarge in public over a method that would be certain to be suggestive of starvation, where food was supposed to be of the greatest importance.

My sick-room success failed to enable me to draw larger checks; but the satisfaction of going into the rooms of the sick and not having to rack my mind over what medicine to give, what food to be taken, was a great compensation for the absence of a large bank account. Professional attainments and abilities play only a small part in the mere business side of the medical profession. An innocent public believes with intense convictions in the efficacy of dosage; and with distorted vision, as the famous knight of La Mancha, sees giants in professional healers who are really only windmills, with whom personal contact in the sick-room is only too often a danger measured by its closeness.

Think of the wasting of the body during sickness; of the brain system, which is life itself, that does not waste: think of the cases of recovery in which for weeks no food is possible for stomach reasons; of the more frequent cases in which recoveries take place after weeks of such scant food as not to be taken into account as a support to vital power by minds governed by reason. Think how disease, in proportion to its severity, is a loss of digestive power, and with cure energy entirely of the brain, how serious a matter it is to lessen it by waste of energy in forcing decomposing food masses through a digestive channel nearly two rods long, food masses that the brain will have none of, and that do not save the fat and muscles; think of all this physiology, and raise this question: "Is this man alone in his faith and practice, or is Nature so in line with him that the entire medical profession is wrong in their dosings and feedings?"

I conclude these cases with an illustration. Think of all this enforced feeding, of the doses to relieve, of the wasting of brain power, and compare with the following illustration, in which case no food was taken for thirty-six days, and yet it was possible for the patient to be about during the greater part of the time.

NOTE.--In this case severe indigestion and nervous troubles and almost daily headaches had been a torture for years. On the morning of the thirty-sixth day, on which the photograph was taken, a visit to the dentist for the extraction of a tooth revealed no fear, as had formerly been the case. Eating was resumed on the thirty-eighth day with no inconvenience. Since then (over six months ago) no trace of the former troubles has reappeared. Loss of weight about twenty pounds.

V.

"Physician, heal thyself!" There is a world of sarcasm in these three words; for about the only advantage the physician has over the laity is that he can do his own dosing. As a general fact, he does no more to prevent bodily ailings than other people, and is just as liable to become the victim of bad habits.

It is my impression that, in proportion, as many physicians become the slaves of tobacco, opium in some form, and alcoholics as are to be found in any other class of people; they are quite as likely to be the victims of various chronic ailings as other people, and with equal impotency to relieve. Every day I see physicians going to the homes of the sick with cigars on fire, signals of the brain system in distress undergoing the lullaby of nicotine; going into rooms where the purest air of heaven ought to prevail, as animated tobacco-signs.

Where is there virtue in this world that is of any practical good whose vital force is not to be found in example rather than in precept? Who has more need to go into the room of the sick with the purest breath, the cleanest tongue, the brightest eyes, the purest complexion, the most radiant countenance, and with a soul free from the bonds of ailings or habits that offend and disable, than the physician? Where is the logic of employing the sick to feed the sick? Is not that a sick doctor whose nerves are so full of plaints as to need the frequent soothings only found in a cigar, that also sears the nerves of taste? Is he not very sick when those nerves require the stronger alcoholic?

There is contagion in good health and sound morals, when daily illustrated, no less than in courage and fear. No physician can be at his best in the rooms of the sick if he be under any bondage from disease or habit.

"Physician, heal thyself!" Physician, how does it happen that you have need to be healed, and of what worth are you if you can neither prevent disease nor cure yourself with your dosings? What availeth it to a man to talk righteously when virtue is not in him?

Ailings, habits blunt all the special senses and the finer instincts and tastes, and impair the power to reason clearly, to infer correctly, to conclude wisely. Only the well have that hopefulness that comes from power in reserve, power that is not wasted through acquired disease and acquired habits. The contagion of health is a power no less than courage or fear.

That man, self-poised, void of fear, General Grant, crushed the Rebellion with a single sentence, "I will fight it out on this line if it takes all summer." That sentence made every man in his army a Grant in courage and confidence. Grant in his prime could puff his cigar while commanding all the armies of his country; but the cigar ultimately destroyed his life, and there was no physician to interpose to prevent one of the most torturing of deaths.

Where is the logic of the sick trying to heal the sick? This question will be more frequently asked in that time to come when the drug-store annex to the sick-room will be much smaller than is now thought necessary.

Human expression is studied in the rooms of the sick as nowhere else; and if the lines are not obscured by the fogs and clouds of disease the signs can be much more clearly distinguished.

A man is now under my care whose soul is of the largest mould, and who is so supremely endowed by reason of intellect, varied tastes and acquirements, as to make life on earth well worth living. His long chronic local ailment has not impaired his power to read me for signs of hope as it seems to me I have never been read before; and never before have I so felt the need to enter a room of the sick with a larger stock of general health. For the time I seem to him to be holding before his eyes the keys of life or death.

The physician should be able to go into the room of the sick to see with clearest vision whatever is revealed to the natural eye; and no less to see with eyes of understanding that he may be an interpreter of conditions that indicate recovery or death. He is the historian of disease, and therefore before he can write he must see clearly all that can be known about the process of cure as revealed by symptoms.

The eye is at its best only in perfect health no less than the reason, the judgment, and the spirits. A few years ago a drouth of many weeks occurred;

in some meadows and pastures the grass seemed dead, beyond the possibility of growth. Every shade of the green had departed; but warm rains came, and in a few days there was a green carpet plush-like in its softness and delicacy.

So the progress of cure may be read on the tongue, on the skin, in the eyes, where there are both eyesight and insight to see and to study.

VI.

For many years I entered the rooms of the sick a sick man myself; I was the victim of that monster of hydraheads, dyspepsia, or, to call it by a more modern title, indigestion.

In my later teens my stomach began seriously to complain over its tasks, and a pint of the essence of bitterness was procured to restore it to power. My mouth was filled with teeth of the sweet kind; hence my horror for the doses far exceeded the milder protests of the stomach. Not the slightest benefit came from my medicinal sufferings, and this ended all routine treatment of my stomach. My intense aversion to the flavor of strong medicines caused me to inflict them as rarely as possible upon other mouths during the drug period of my practice.

Mine seemed to be a weary stomach, in which the tired sense was a close approach to acute pain for hours after each meal. When a medical student I found nothing in the books, in the advice of my preceptor, nor in the lectures at the university, but what proposed to cure me through drugs that were abhorrent. As I never encountered any cures nor received the slightest benefit from my experiments, I was deterred from injuring myself through persistent dosage.

In the early part of my student career I was behind a drug-counter, where I had ample experience in putting up prescriptions, and had an excellent opportunity to measure medical men as revealed in their formulas and the results in many cases in which failure was the rule in chronic ailings; and I was not encouraged to abuse myself through the results as revealed by any form of medication.

For the benefit of those who suffer from complainings of the stomach I give a condensed summing-up of myself. I was born with a wiry constitution, but of the lean kind, and a weak stomach, the chiefest ancestral legacy. With ability to see with intense sense very much to enjoy in this world, my resources in this way were boundless, hence I was always full of hope and cheer.

All the senses of my palate were of the acute kind, and so were a continual source of the penalties of gluttony. Whatever else there might be alack with me, there was never a lack of appetite. I was able to eat at each meal food enough which, if fully digested, would have redeemed the wastes of any day of labor; and not only this, but also enough of sugar-enticing foods to anticipate the wastes of the following day.

Growing up in the country and with an intense fondness for the tart sweetness of apples, pears, and peaches, and the harmlessness of eating them no matter how full the stomach with hearty food, without question my stomach was never void of pomace during the entire fruit season.

Whenever I sat down to eat there was an onrush of all the senses of the palate as the outrush of imprisoned children to the ecstatic activities of the school-yard; hence over-eating always, with never a sense of satiety. The penalties were realized in painful digestion, with the duodenum the chiefest of protesting voices.

A time came when gas would so accumulate as to make the heart labor from mere pressure, the inevitable insufficiency of breath causing a lack of a 雛ation of the blood. With a constant waste of power in the stomach there was always a sense of weariness; hence I was never able to know the luxury of power in reserve. All through life my best efforts were the result of intellectual inebriation, with always corresponding exhaustion as the direct result. This weakness compelled me to waste the least time on people who could not interest me, and to spend much time alone to recharge my exhausted batteries.

For such a case as mine there is not to-day to be found an intelligent hint in any medical text-book as to the physiological way to recovery.

The breakfasts in my house were of a character that, without ham, sausage, eggs, steaks, or chops, they would not have been considered worth spending time over. I had reached a time when a general collapse seemed to be impending; but it was stayed for a few years by the new life that came to me through the evolutions of health in the rooms of the sick that seemed to portend possible professional glories: but as the years went on I suffered more and more from nervous prostration through waste of power in the stomach.

My friends began to enlarge upon my wretched looks, and with no little concern; but none were wise enough to realize that my need was for words that reminded of life and not of death.

By chance I met an old friend on the street when he happened to be thinking about ways in daily food in Europe, from which he had just returned, and at once he began to talk, not about my wretched looks, but about the exceedingly light breakfasts customary in all the great centres where he had been. They consisted only of a roll and a cup of coffee. I was impressed just enough not to forget the fact, but without there being a hint in it to set me to thinking.

But the time came, "the fulness of time." There came a morning when for the first time I remembered that when in ordinary health I had no desire to breakfast; but there was a sense of such general exhaustion from power wasted over an unusual food mass not needed at the previous evening meal that my morning coffee was craved as the morning dram by the chronic toper. Only this, and a forenoon resulted of such comfort of body, such cheer, and such mental and physical energy as had never been realized since my young manhood was happy in the blessed unconsciousness of having a stomach that, no matter how large or how numerous the daily meals, never complained.

As for the dinner that followed, it was taken with an acuteness of relish and was handled with a power of digestion that were also a new, rich experience; but the afternoon fell far short of the forenoon. The experience was so remarkable that I at once gave up all eating in the morning, and with such reviving effects upon all my powers that the results began to be noticed by all friends.

So originated the no-breakfast plan. Up to this time I had never had a thought of advising anyone to do without food when desired; much less that any of the three daily meals should be given up. My war was against feeding when acute sickness had abolished all desire for food, and this I had been able to conduct many years without exciting suspicion of a general practice of homicide.

The improvement in my own case was so instant and so marked that I began to advise the same to others, and with the result that each would make known the redeeming work to suffering friends, and so the idea spread in a friend-to-friend way.

Now the American breakfast, in point of sheer necessity, is believed to be the most important meal of the day, as the means for strength that is to be called out for the forenoon of labor, and believed with a force of insistence that warrants a conclusion that a night of sleep is more exhausting to all the powers than the day of labor.

To go into the fresh air, to do anything with an empty stomach, is to invite a fainting by the way, is the general impression; but there were scarcely any cases in which there was not sufficient improvement to prevent all possibility of a return to the heavy breakfasts that had been abandoned.

How did this scheme affect me in a professional way, that is, in the reputation as a physician of average balance of brain functions? Some of my professional brethren of strong conviction and ready command of language began at once to try to abolish the dangerous heresy by suggesting that on this one subject I was absolutely crazy. Of course, their patrons took up this idea with avidity; and so there was a babble of tongues, with myself the central point of attack as crank-in-chief of all cranks. This is not the language of exaggeration; for whatever the law and modern civilization permitted to abolish me professionally was inflicted with tongues by the thousands, the war being made all the more exciting and interesting by the enthusiasm of new recruits to the heresy from the professional domains of my medical brethren.

What did I gain by this professionally? Mostly the odium of heresy during the first few years; but with it was the supreme satisfaction that came from seeing more additions to bright eyes and happy faces than medicine ever gave, and in a way that would redound to my own good at some time. The fact is, that as a means to better health, no matter what nor where the disease, there is no limit to its application. As a universal panacea its powers are matchless.

For a time I saw no farther than a cure of stomach condition and resulting general comfort. That any disease was to be cured otherwise than in the stomach by means so simple, did not occur as an original conception; but the fact that giving up the morning meal was attended with improvement of all local diseases set me to thinking. Many of my patients became thin under the regime; but as this was attended by an increase of strength, not even the alarm of anxious friends without faith was ever able to induce a return fully to the old ways.

But how explain the loss of weight? A clue came from the following case: The first-born of a young mother had an habitual diarrhoea from birth lasting many months; and yet it seemed well nourished, for it was unusually fat and heavy for its age; but the days and nights were long in the care of this apparently well-nourished child. The symptoms were heedless to the every-hour dosing of pellets, or from the tumblers of apparently purest water.

Now this mother, young as she was, was a woman of convictions, and with courage to follow each to an ultimate conclusion. She had heard of miracles resulting from only three feedings per day during the nursing period; and so, notwithstanding a storm of opposition from a vast circle of relatives, she put this first-born rigidly on the three-meal plan, with the result of immediate cessation of the bowel trouble, but with rapid decline in weight.

This caused anxiety, and I was called upon for advice. In every respect except the weight-loss the improvement was wonderful. After much thought there was a sudden flash of the truth: there were an abnormal weight and bulk, due to the general dropsy of debility, similar in character to the swelling of the feet and limbs in the old and feeble. The thickened walls of the bloodvessels, toned with health, caused absorption; but the eyes of the friends would not open to the miracle for a very long time, and so render justice to the heroine, the young mother. As an aider and abettor of such a flagrant system of starvation, I had my full share of opprobrium; but, aided by the strong-minded, sensible mother, Nature gained a sweeping victory, and thus this case cleared my mind from confusion as to the anomaly.

One of my medical friends with whom calomel was as a sheet-anchor often asserted that babies would actually get fat on it. That bulk would actually increase by use of the forceful medicine is likely; but that the increase would be dropsical I think is unquestionable.

The dropsy of debility is due to a loss of tone of the vascular system; the walls of the vessels become thinner and therefore dilate. In the feet and limbs of the old and greatly enfeebled by disease the veins become distended to abnormal size by the force of gravity, resulting in effusion of water into the cellular tissues, which increases when in the upright position during the day and decreases when in the horizontal position at night.

A toning up of the entire vascular system, by which a reverse current from the tissues into the bloodvessels is made possible, is the only means for relief.

This flash-light upon the part physics plays in the cure of disease put me upon the true lines of investigation, and furnished a key for the solution of many problems. From this time on I was to be kept busy, not in winning victories, but in studying them.

This new physiology was not fully apprehended until long after the no-breakfast plan was taken up. It came to me link by link; but the missing link was the fact that food only restores waste, that lost strength is only restored by sleep; and it now seems to me that I was very dull not to have found it out long before I did. It seems to me that no method of health culture, none in the treatment of disease can have any physiological basis where these facts are not taken into account.

For a time I failed to look beyond the ailments of the stomach for curative results, until really surprising news began to reach me from many sources. There would come to me those who had to tell about clearer vision, acuter hearing, a stronger sense of smelling, etc., senses that were not thought to be affected by disease; or there would be news that chronic, local ailings, as nasal or bronchial catarrhs, skin diseases, hemorrhoids, or other intractable disease, in some mysterious manner, were undergoing a decline under the new regime.

In the domain of drugs we have medicines that vivid imagination has endowed with presumed affinities for locations that are diseased. They enter the circulation and happily get off at the right spot, to act curatively; but no theories are advanced as to how they aid in the construction of new cells or atoms, or how they aid in the disposal of the old ones.

Construction, destruction! There is no death of atoms: really nothing is generated, nothing destroyed: the change is but the rearranging of ultimate elements; and how is a drug to influence any more than would be in case of the affinities of chemistry?

Hazy conceptions, crude means! The ultimate cell multiplies by division to become bone, nails, hair, ligaments, muscles, fat, the brain, the whole body. Where along the line in the reconstructive work called by a disease or injury is a medicine to apply with power to aid? In what way the need to be expressed, in what operative way the helpful assistance made clear, that faith without works that are seen can be made strong?

The chemist never rushes into print with news that another element has been discovered until demonstrative evidence has placed the matter beyond all question. If anything new is discovered in the firmaments, adequate means to an end will be able to reveal it to all interested eyes.

The impressions of science are quite different from the impressions of the materia medica; and the miracles of cure that are displayed by the column in even the highest class public prints are never in reach of scientific explanation.

A new element is announced; we know instantly that it has been actually discovered. A new cure is announced; we instantly may know that the evidences will never be displayed along the lines of science.

I now unfold a theory of my own of the origin and development of disease, and the development of cure, in which the physical changes involved in some of the processes are in reach of the microscope.

It is my impression that, with rare exceptions, people are born with actual structural weaknesses, local or general, that may be called ancestral legacies. These are known as constitutional tendencies to disease.

In parts structurally weak at birth the bloodvessels, because of thin and weak walls, are larger than in normal parts, and because of dilatation the blood circulates slower. There is an undue pressure upon all between-vessel structures, a pressure that must lessen the nutrient supply more or less, according to its degree. The death of parts in boils and abscesses is due, I believe, to strangulation of the nerve-supply. The bloodvessels are elastic, and capable of contraction and dilatation, a matter regulated by the brain.

Now in these weaknesses always lie the possibilities of disease; they may be supposed the weak links in the constitutional chain, and can no more be made stronger than the constitutional design than can the body as a whole. By whatever means brain power is lessened abnormality is incited in the weak parts; hence gradually from the original weakness there is a summing up, as a bronchial or nasal catarrh, or other acute or chronic local or general disease.

The first step in any disease is the impression that lessens brain power; the slightest depressing emotion, the slightest sense of discomfort, lessens brain power, and to a like degree the tone of all the bloodvessels; hence dilatation in degree. That the stomach, as the most abused organ of the body, plays the largest part in over-drafts upon the brain is not a matter of doubt.

Let us develop a chronic disease along these lines, with nasal catarrh for an illustration. As tone is regulated entirely by the brain system, all taxing of the brain increases the debility of the nasal structures. In course of time the debility so increases through whatever also debilitates the brain, that a stage is reached when water in the blood begins to escape through the thin walls of the vessels and mingles with the natural secretion of the membrane, and a catarrhal discharge is the result. In severe cases a time may be reached when death of parts from the strangling pressure may occur, and then we have an ulcerative catarrh.

This evolution will go on as determined by the gravity of the ancestral weakness, by the natural strength of the dynamo, the brain, and the severity of the debilitating forces to which it may be subjected.

No one is ever attacked by a nasal or any other catarrh, nor by any other chronic ailings. They all start from structural weaknesses that are inherited, and they are the evolutionary results of brain-wearying forces.

If a specialist were asked to express the actual condition of a diseased structure that seems to call for medicinal aid, and to tell just how medicated sprays, washes, and douches are to reach all the parts involved, with healing power, and in what way that power is exercised--in other words, what work actually is to be done, and how medicine is to do it--he would not be able to enlighten his questioner no matter how fertile his conception, how dexterous his use of language. In fact, the healing power of drugs exists in fertile imaginations rather than among those ultimate processes where disease is cured, where disease destroys.

As the care moves by the power evolved in the dynamo, so do the bloodvessels contract and relax as determined by brain conditions. Dilating bloodvessels, effusion of water from thinning walls, the between-vessels starving pressure, increasing general debility of all the structures involved-- this is the gradual evolution of catarrh and of all other chronic diseases.

From this it was seen that no form of local treatment can avail to relieve the operative cause in cases of this kind. Tone must be added to all the weakened, dilated vessels, in order to contract and thicken their walls so as to stop the leakage, and to relieve that pressure upon the between structures that have become an 鎚 ic through lack of nourishment.

That an evolution in reverse is the one need scarcely calls for argument. It is the brain that needs our attention, and we meet its need by saving its rare powers from wasting.

We will do this by cutting down, as far as possible, all the activities for which it furnishes power, even as we would diminish the number of cars where power in the dynamo had become deficient; we will either sever the wires that connect with the stomach, or make a marked reduction in the labor to be performed in the stomach. With power accumulating in the brain, power will reach the utmost recesses of debility and disease, with Nature to do all the healing.

To reinforce this physiology, this statement may be made with the strongest emphasis: the medical treatment of chronic disease fails inevitably because it fails to consider the vital force involved. The brain has no part in the treatment of chronic disease by the specialist, where drugs are a means to an end never reached: there are only a disappointment and an interchange of pocket-books.

In all parts suffering with pain there is congestion, swelling. The bloodvessels are distended; hence the nerves suffer violence in stretching or from pressure. The pain simply adds to the abnormal conditions by causing an active determination of the blood to the involved parts. To relieve pain, then, is curative, because it lessens the abnormal congestion.

The no-breakfast plan with me proved a matter of life unto life. With my morning coffee there were forenoons of the highest physical energy, the clearest condition of mind, and the acutest sense of everything enjoyable.

The afternoons were always in marked sluggishness by contrast, from the taxing of digestion.

Without realizing that the heavy meals of the day were a tax upon the brain, I would scarcely get away from the table before I began to feel more generally tired out than the severest taxing from a long forenoon of general activity ever made me. With the filled stomach, fatigue, general exhaustion, came as a sudden attack rather than as an evolution from labor, and there would be several hours of unfitness for doing any kind of service well.

In the application of this method to others I had the great satisfaction of good results without any exceptions; and the missionary work was begun by friends among friends, fairly spreading better health and adding thereby more and more disaster to my name.

More and more I became a focus of adverse criticism in all matters where level-headedness was deemed important. My acute cases began to be watched with hostile interest, as if homicide from starvation were the inevitable result in all cases. My country had become the country of an enemy.

Not being able to give my patients clearly defined reasons for the general and local improvements resulting from a forenoon fast as a method in hygiene, it had to be spread from relieved persons to suffering friends; and according to the need, the sufferers from various ailings would be willing to try anything new where efforts through the family physician or patent medicines had completely failed; it was spread as if by contagion, among the failures of the medical profession.

Among those to become interested at an early date was a prominent minister who wore the title of D. D., and for a time his interest was intense. He came to me one day with word that a member of his household, well known to me as a young woman of unusual ability and culture, had not been able to take solid food at his table for a year, and he believed that my treatment would avail in her case. To this she was very averse, since every treatment her hapless stomach had received had only added to the debility, until disability had become the result. She finally came to me to be relieved from the forceful importunity of her reverend friend, who had excited my eager interest with a prophecy that unusual literary distinction would follow a cure, as there were abilities of the very highest order, in his estimation.

She came, and I had no difficulty in securing such a vacation for the worn-out stomach that it could begin with solid food when the time to eat arrived. The vacation was so brief and power had accumulated so rapidly that almost any food could be taken without discomfort, and no trouble ever came not invited by a relapse from the better way of living that had really created a new stomach.

This case caused more notoriety over the no-breakfast plan than any that ever occurred in the city. As a writer of biographies and of articles in high-class journals and magazines, this talented woman has been a miracle of patient, persistent study and investigation.

This endorsement in high places greatly added to my reputation as a physician with distorted mind, for the idea that any good could come from a short fast, to be followed by the giving up of that needed morning meal, was too absurd for sober reflection, too violently revolutionary to be even patiently considered.

The no-breakfast plan was not so very long in becoming known over the entire city; a bridge had been crossed, and every plank taken up and destroyed; thence the ways into new families were nearly closed.

I am enlarging a little upon the opposition that met me from all points, because all who are to be convinced that these are the true ways in health culture will begin at once to enlighten their ailing friends, and will, therefore, encounter the same opposition. "Sir, you have not had enough opposition," said bluff, old Samuel Johnson. There will be no need to complain of any lack of this kind in the efforts to render suffering friends the only aid possible, that will be in persistent efforts of Nature.

My medical brethren considered the scheme only as they would consider an invasion of smallpox or a heresy whose methods were a danger to life. One physician, a woman specialist, informed me that she was continually importuned as to her professional opinion of the new craze that had invaded the city. That all other physicians were equally called upon, that they would condemn, was inevitable; and I permitted them the largest liberty without the least resentment; but there was the sustaining cheer of seeing the happiest faces that only increased as the heresy spread.

My attendance upon the severely sick became more taxing because of the exceeding concern in the immediate environment, that the pangs of starvation were being added to the pangs of disease.

As none of my professional brethren ever manifested any desire to be enlightened on this subject, I did not volunteer, since I felt the wiser way would be to wait an adequate amount of evidence before making any public announcements of presumed important discoveries in practical hygiene.

My experiences in the rooms of the sick had convinced me, long before I gave up my morning meal, that death from starvation was so remote as practically to exclude it from consideration; hence with the great improvement that was the immediate result in my own case I could from the first speak with a "thus saith the Lord" emphasis on the safety of going through a forenoon "on an empty stomach."

As no one could come into my office without my being able to give the assurance of at least some relief that would be immediately realized, that would be felt even to the finger-ends, my office became more and more a lecture-room, a school of health culture for the education of missionaries, for a friend-to-friend uplifting into higher life.

All I needed for my own sake was that missing link to clothe my words with all the desired power. With so much to enliven, to encourage, it was as if I were sitting at the very feet of Nature, so thrilled by her wonderful stories that I was utterly unconscious of the storm of ridicule and epithet to which I was subjected.

Once in a while Nature would favor me with a miracle in the way of an inspiring change. A man in the early prime of life had reached a condition in which he habitually rejected every breakfast. Two trips to Europe and a year in the hands of a Berlin specialist for the stomach failed to relieve; and yet he was not so disabled as to prevent him attending to his ordinary business affairs; the stomach seemed to be eccentric in being merely irritable without structural disease.

I asked him if he felt that the breakfasts which would not stay down were doing him any good. To this he had to assent that they were not. I told him if the breakfast only to result in a heave-offering were omitted he would be better able for his duties of the forenoon. He began at once to raise his brows.

It was not difficult for him to see that if no breakfasts were put into his stomach none would have to be thrown up with sickening effort, and hence he could not but be better for the forenoon services if the sick spell were omitted. The fact was, the breakfast would soon be rejected, and then the hours of rest would enable the stomach to handle the dinner without the repetition of the morning sickness.

Only a few words from me of this kind, and thence on there were no breakfasts; and from the first all the complaints from the stomach ceased, and he used to remark that he began to get well as soon as I began to talk to him.

Now this man with his family was a recent arrival in this city, and his first intimate acquaintance was one who had been relieved of weekly headaches of a skull-bursting kind through the no-breakfast plan--thus the missionary contagion.

For many years I was content to allow people to have the morning coffee or tea as desired, with the largest liberty of dinner gluttony; and this was really the only means possible for the introduction of an innovation so radical. To have given nothing to relieve the morning want for something in the stomach to set the wheels of life in motion would have been a failure from the first. With all the coffee break of the fast was attended by so marked an increase of cheer and general strength, and the enjoyment of the general meal at or before noon was so immeasurably increased, that the method spread as a contagion against which professional denouncement and ridicule were in vain.

And with all converts I found that the experiences in the penalties of gluttony were so enlightening, so restraining, that there was apparently little need to say much more as to the quantity or quality of food, what and how to eat.

The enthusiasm of all over the forenoons of power and comfort, to be followed by a luxury of meals never before realized, fully satisfied my pride in professional success; and all the more because the penalties of gluttony were seldom charged to my account.

It was only after the missing link was found and added to the chain that I could fully realize the enormous waste of strength and the mental and moral degradation from eating food in excess, because the enticements of relish are taken for the actual needs of the body. Think of it! Actual soul power involved in ridding the stomach and bowels of the foul sewage of food in excess, food in a state of decomposition, to be forced through nearly two rods of bowels and largely at the expense of the soul itself!!

Oh, gluttony, with its jaws of death, its throat an ever-open gate to the stomach of torment!

VII.

When I finally arrived at a point of vision where I could see the stomach as a mere machine, that it could no more act without brain-power than brawny arms with their nerves severed could wield a sledge, I began a study of digestion with new interest, with a view to save power from undue waste.

It is the sense of relish, of flavor, that is behind all the woes of indigestion, and not the sense of hunger. The sweetened foods; the pies, cakes, puddings, etc., that are eaten merely from a sense of relish after the sense of hunger has become fully sated, and generally by far more of the plainer foods than waste demands, is the wrecking sin at all but the humblest tables.

Rapid eating, by which there is imperfect solution of the tougher solids and a filling of the stomach before the hunger sense can naturally be appeased, is the additional evil to insure serious consequences to the stomach and brain.

For merely practical purposes, all that is necessary to know about the digestive process is that by a peculiar arrangement of the muscle forces of the stomach the food is made to revolve in such a way as to wipe the exuding digestive juice from the walls; that, therefore, the finer the division of the solids by mastication the more rapid the solution to the absorbing condition. That meat in finer particles will sooner dissolve than meat in large, solid masses is clearly seen.

It will be recalled that digestive conditions are really soul conditions, as if there were actual wires extending from the very depths of the soul itself to each individual gland, with power to ebb and flow as the mental condition shall determine.

It may be presumed that power to digest is the power to revolve food in the stomach and the power to generate the gastric juice as determined by the power of the brain, the glands themselves not holding their juice in mere reserve, but power to generate in reserve. Thus it is seen that food in excess is in every way exhaustive as the immediate result.

These may be called the subjective conditions of digestion. Now let us consider some of the objective conditions from the standpoint of moral science. What the sunshine of a warm day is to all growing things on the earth, so is that shining seen in other faces that reaches the depths of the human soul with brightness and life.

Overeating is so universal from the general ignorance of practical physiology that few stomachs have a time for a full clearing with the needed rest before the time of another filling arrives. It is therefore a matter of sheer necessity not only to attain and maintain the utmost possible cheer of soul, but it is also a necessity to have cheer in other souls with whom relations are intimate.

As a matter of extraneous digestive aid, a cheerful soul in a family is an abiding source of digestive energy to all in social contact. It affects the digestive energy of all, as the breeze the fire, as the clearing sky the low spirits from the gloom of chill and fogs. The eyes that do not glisten with higher life, the lines upon the face that are not alive with cheerful, kindly emotions, the frowning look, the word that cuts deeply, have their repressive effects upon digestive energy within their remorseless reach.

The moral science of digestive energy is a new study; it is not known as a factor in the process of digestion; but the time is coming when cheer of soul will become a study as of one of the finer arts, and then human homes will not be so much like lesser lunatic asylums without the restraining hands of a wise superintendent.

Life will be different in homes when all within the age of reason shall realize that their words without kindness, their looks without cheer, are forces that tend to physical and moral degradation, really nothing less than death-dealing energies upon all lives within their reach. The power of human kindness has ever been a favorite theme with the moralist, but it has not been considered with reference to its power upon digestion.

Anger is mental and moral chaos; it is insanity; it is revenge in the fury of a hurricane; and sensitive natures have the greatest need for the largest measure of health in order that these human tempests shall be under larger restraint.

The gloomy, the irritable, the dyspeptic Christian is a dispenser of death and not of the higher life, and his religious faith does not spread by the contagiousness of example: and because of the solemnity, of the exceeding importance of his sense of the possibilities of the life beyond death he has all the more need to have that physical and moral strength that his daily walk, conversation, and mien may be consistent, forceful, and uplifting.

To this great end study, study to see cheer everywhere, and above all things to possess it. Good health is also contagious, and, no less than disease, has a reflex impression. Only above the chill dampness, the fogs, and clouds is the clear sky with the blazing sun. There are undreamed-of possibilities of getting above the worriments of life through an intelligent understanding and application of the physiology of cheer as the chief force in the life of the body, mind, and soul.

VIII.

Having finally arrived at the conviction that from the first wink in the morning until the last at night strength departs, not in any way to be kept up by food, that from the last wink at night until the first in the morning strength returns, I became fully endowed to tell all the sick and afflicted in the most forceful way that with the strength of the brain recharged by sleep is all the labor of the day performed, and that no labor is so taxing upon human muscles that it cannot be performed longer without fatigue when the breakfast is omitted.

That this is possible came to me as a great surprise and in this way: a farmer with a large assortment of ailments came to me for relief through drugs. He was simply advised to take coffee mornings, rest mainly during forenoons, and when a normal appetite and power to digest would come he would be able to work after resuming his breakfasts. This man, who was more than fifty years old, was the first manual laborer to be advised to observe a morning fast.

Several months after, he came to me with news that his ailing had all departed, and that he had been able to do harder work on his coffee breakfasts than ever before with breakfasts of solids. And if he so worked with power during forenoons, why not others? Why not all?

This no-breakfast plan was so contagious that I was not long in finding that farmers in all directions were beginning to go to their labors with much less food in their stomachs than had been their wont, and in all cases with added power of muscle.

Only recently three farmers went into the field one hot morning to cradle oats, the most trying of all work on the farm; two of them had their stomachs well filled with hearty foods. With profuse sweating and water by the quart because of the chemical heat arising from both digestion and decomposition, these toiled through the long hours with much weariness. The third man had all his strength for the swinging of the cradle, the empty stomach not even calling for water; with the greatest ease he kept his laboring friends in close company and when the noon hour came he was not nearly so tired as they.

A man who had been a great sufferer from indigestion, a farmer, found such an increase of health and strength from omitting the morning meal that he became able to cradle rye, a much heavier grain than oats, during an entire forenoon "on an empty stomach." Later he went from one December to the following April on one daily meal, and not only with ease, but with a gain in weight in addition. During these months this man did all the work usual in farm-houses, besides riding several hours over a milk route during the forenoons.

In this city resides a carpenter, formerly subject to frequent sicknesses, who for the past five years has walked nearly a mile to the shop where he is employed without even as much as a drink of water for breakfast; and this not only without any sicknesses, but with an increase in weight of fifteen pounds also.

More than a dozen years ago a farmer who was not diseased in any way, but who had been in the habit of eating three times a day at a well-spread table, and at mid-forenoon taking a small luncheon for hunger-faintness, omitted his breakfast and morning luncheon, and has been richly rewarded since then in escaping severe colds and other ailings. He conclusively felt that his forenoon was the better half of the day for clear-headedness and hard labor; he has added nearly a score of pounds to his weight, and his case has been a wonder to all his farmer friends, who see only starvation in cutting down brain and needless stomach taxing.

I must now ask the reader to bear with me while I apply the principles of this new hygiene with a good deal of reiteration, trying to vary them in utterance as far as possible. The need of daily food is primarily a matter of waste and supply, the waste always depending upon the amount of loss through the general activities, manual labor being the most destructive.

Across the street from where I live a new house is being built: for many days during the chilly, windy month of March several men have been engaged high in the air, handling green boards, studs, and joists for ten hours each day; and yet these men are not eating more food daily than hundreds of brain-workers who never have general exercise. The workmen across the street eat to satisfy hunger; the brain-workers, to satisfy the sense of relish; and the meals of the latter are habitually in excess of the real demands because of wasted bodies.

In spite of the apparent overeating of the brain-worker, I believe the farmer and the manual laborer break down at an earlier age, for the reason that they overwork and generally eat when too tired to digest fully: the farmer is rarely content to do one day's work in one day when the crop season invites him to make the most of fair days.

With successes rapidly multiplying in all directions within my circuit, the desire became urgent for some way to make my new hygiene known to the public. My first thought was to get some eminent divine interested through a cure that would compel him to a continual talk as to how he became saved.

At a great denominational meeting in Chicago I chanced to hear a splendid address from a sallow-faced professor of a divinity school, the Rev. Dr. G. W. N.; and after a great deal of reflection I resolved, without consulting him, to write him a series of letters on health culture, hoping that he would become so immediately interested as to permit me a complete unfolding of my theory and practice.

I began the series, taking all the chances to be considered a crank; they were continued until the end without response, when later I received a brief note with sarcasm in every line. At least my letters had been read; for he informed me that he had no confidence in my theory, giving me a final summing up with his estimate that there were more "cranks" in the medical profession than in any other. I was not in the least cast down at this long-range estimate, since I had become quite used to close-at-hand ridicule.

There was before me the unknown time when a still more eminent D. D. would both accept and practise my theory, and also give the world his estimate in an elaborate preface to a book that in the fulness of time the ways opened to me to write and have published.

I was sent for by a man who had become a moral and physical wreck, his body being reduced to nearly a skeleton condition from consumption. As he was taking an average of two quarts of whiskey per week, I accepted the charge of his case with reluctance.

I was not able in any way to change his symptoms for the better; there had been no hint of hunger for many weeks, and the mere effort to swallow or even taste the most tempting dainties was painful to witness. He was taken with a severe pain in his side, which was fully relieved with the hypodermic needle, and there followed several hours of general comfort and no desire for the alcoholic. Seeing this I was strongly impressed that by continuing the dosings for a time the seared stomach might get into a better condition and the fast be followed by a natural hunger.

This is what actually followed: in about a week the dosings were reduced to mere hints, and without any desire for stimulants there came a desire for broiled steak and baked potatoes, which were taken with great relish. Thence on this was mainly the bill of fare, and the half-filled bottle remained on his table untouched, undesired; and in time there were added more than a score of pounds to his wasted body.

Now it chanced that this regenerative work was seen day after day by his friend, who was badly in need of an all-round treatment to meet the needs of his case; he was a man of keen intellect, of real ability of both mind and muscle. Becoming deeply interested in the theory behind the miracle he saw unfolding day after day, and all the more because of a total extinction of the drink-habit that was deep seated through long duration, he began to omit his morning meals.

He saw more than his own case. He had been a manager of book agencies, and when he found also his desire for the cigar undergoing a rapid decline, he became possessed with the idea that a book might be written on the subject. The time came when he could sit down in the office of the Henry Bill

Publishing Company, Norwich, Conn., a picture of health, to interview Mr. Charles C. Haskell on the subject of publishing a book. Mr. Haskell had known him in less healthful years, and he marvelled at the change.

I had duly suggested, and with great emphasis, that no publisher would listen to him unless he were sick enough to be interested in the theory and would give a test by actual trial. He found Mr. Haskell in very low health. Experts had sent him on a tour through Europe in search of that health he failed to find; his body was starving on three meals a day that were not digested, and he began to arrange his affairs with reference to a near-at-hand breakdown.

To this man was made such an appeal as men are rarely able to make, because a regenerated life was also vocal in utterance. To him a miracle seemed to have been wrought, and he listened to each word as if to a reprieve from a death seemingly inevitable.

As there was no disease of the stomach, it required only a few days for Mr. Haskell to acquire so much of new life that he felt as one born again, and a week had not passed before I had his earnest request to put my hygiene into a book, he taking all chances of failure.

He began to advise all ailing friends to give up their breakfasts or to fast until natural hunger came, getting many marvellous results. One of his first thoughts was to have the forthcoming book introduced by some eminent divine who could write through the inspiration of experience.

In a visit to Norwich of that evangelist of world-wide eminence, George F. Pentecost, D. D., then of London, Eng., the opportunity came, and for a case of "special conversion" he was made the guest of Mr. Haskell. He was easily persuaded to the system, and his need is expressed in the following from the introduction of The True Science of Living, which was actually written without his having read a single line of the manuscript.

"Taking the theory upon which this system of living is based into account-- and even to my lay mind it seemed most reasonable--and the testimony which I personally received from both men and women, delicate and biliously strong, workingmen, merchants, doctors, and preachers, delicate ladies for years invalided and in a state of collapse, and some who had never been ill, but were a hundred per cent. better for living without breakfast, I resolved to give up my breakfast. I pleaded at first that it might be my luncheon instead, for I have all my life enjoyed my breakfast more than any other meal. But no! it was the breakfast that must go. So on a certain fine Monday morning I bade farewell to the breakfast-room. For a day or two I suffered slight headaches from what seemed to me was the want of food; but I soon found that they were just the dying pains of a bad habit. After a week had passed I never thought of wanting breakfast; and though I was often present in the breakfast-rooms of friends whom I was visiting, and every tempting luxury of the breakfast was spread before me, I did not desire food at all, feeling no suggestion of hunger. Indeed now, after a few months, the thought of breakfast never occurs to me. I am ready for my luncheon (or breakfast if you please) at one o'clock, but am never hungry before that hour.

"As for the results of this method of living, I can only relate them as I have personally experienced them:

"1. I have not had the first suggestion of a sick headache since I gave up my breakfast. From my earliest boyhood I do not remember ever having gone a whole month without being down with one of these attacks, and for thirty years, during the most active part of my life, I have suffered with them oftentimes, more or less, every day for a month or six weeks at a time, and hardly ever a whole fortnight passed without an acute attack that has sent me to bed or at least left me to drag through the day with intense bodily suffering and mental discouragement.

"2. I have gradually lost a large portion of my surplus fat, my weight having gone down some twenty pounds, and my size being reduced by several inches at the point where corpulency was the most prominent; and I am still losing weight and decreasing in size.

"3. I find that my skin is improving in texture, becoming softer, finer, and more closely knit than heretofore. My complexion and eyes have cleared, and all fulness of the face and the tendency to flushness in the head have disappeared.

"4. I experience no fulness and unpleasantness after eating, as I so often did before. As a matter of fact, though I enjoy my meals (and I eat everything my appetite and taste call for) as never before, eating with zest, I do not think I eat as much as I used to do; but I am conscious of better digestion; my food does not lie so long in my stomach, and that useful organ seems to have gone out of the gas-producing business.

"5. I am conscious of a lighter step and a more elastic spring in all my limbs. Indeed, a brisk walk now is a pleasure which I seek to gratify, whereas before the prescribed walk for the sake of exercise was a horrible bore to me.

"6. I go to my study and to my pulpit on an empty stomach without any sense of loss of strength mentally or physically--on the other hand, with freshness and vigor which is delightful. In this respect I am quite sure that I am in every way advantaged."

Rev. George Sherman Richards, after more than fifteen years of frequent severe headaches that were supposed to be due to heredity, has had entire freedom during the five years of the No-breakfast Plan. He can hardly be surpassed as a picture of perfect health.

One of the first prominent converts who finally surrendered to Mr. Haskell, whose persistence was beyond fatigue, was the editor of the Norwich, Conn., Bulletin, a special friend. There was no want of conviction on his part, but the evil day to begin the morning fast was continually postponed. Finally, one morning when he was specially busy and charged with impatience, the beaming and hopeful face of Mr. Haskell appeared. Said the busy man, "Mr. Haskell, if you will walk right out of that door, I will promise you to begin tomorrow morning to do without breakfasts." Mr. Haskell walked out--the breakfasts were given up, and some years later I was personally informed that he believed that his life had been saved thereby.

One of the expedients was to send a circular about the book to every foreign missionary of every denomination, and as a result one of these fell into the hands of Rev. W. E. Rambo, in India. He had become a mere shadow of his former self from ulcerated bowels, the sequel of a badly treated case of typhoid fever. For seven months there had been daily movements tinged with blood; the appetite was ravenous, and large meals were taken without any complainings from the stomach. Before a well-spread table his desire to eat would become simply furious, and it was indulged regardless of quality and quantity. His brain system had become so exhausted that reason and judgment had no part in this hurricane of hunger.

There were seven successive physicians in this case, some of them with many titles. The first one he called on reaching New England cut his food down to six bland meals daily. All of them had tried to cure the offending ulcers by dosings. Think whether bleeding ulcers on the body would get well with their tender surfaces subjected to the same grinding, scratching process from bowel rubbish!

He was in condition on his arrival to lose six pounds during the first week of six "bland" daily meals. After reading the True Science of Living he discharged his physician and came under my personal care. These ulcers were treated with the idea of giving them the same rest as if each had been the end of a fractured bone. To relieve pain, to hold the bowel still, and to abolish the morbid hunger, a few doses with the hypodermic needle were a seeming necessity.

In less than two weeks this starving man of skin and bones was relieved of all symptoms of disease, and there seemed a moderate desire for food of the nourishing kind. Less than two weeks were required for all those ulcers to become covered with a new membrane: but for full three weeks only those liquid foods were given that had no rubbish in them to prove an irritant to the new, delicate membrane covering the ulcers. For a time after the third week there was only one light daily meal, with a second added when it seemed safe to take it.

In a little more than three months there was a gain of forty-two and a half pounds of flesh, as instinct with new, vigorous life as if freshly formed by the divine hand. My last word from this restored man was after he, his wife, and four children had been back in India for a year and a half, where they were all living on the two-meal plan without any sicknesses, and he had a class of one hundred and sixty native boys on the same plan.

Who can fail to see the science and the sense to relieve all diseases of the digestive tract? There are no cases of hemorrhoids not malignant in character, in which total relief will not be the result if fasts are long enough; no cases of anal fistula that will not finally close if they can have that rest from violence that is their only need; and equally all ulcers and fissures that make life a history of torture.

No case with structural disease of any part of the digestive tract not malignant has yet come under my care in which there has not been a cure, or in which there has not been a cure in sight. Through a fast we may let the diseased parts in the digestive tract rest as we would a broken bone or wound on the body.

Several missionaries have regained health on these new lines, who have returned to preach and practise a larger gospel than before. One returned from the Congo region of Africa with such wreckage of health as to make any active service impossible. Mr. Haskell met him in New York, and in time he returned with twenty-four missionaries, all as converts to the new gospel of health, and to have that sustained health only possible through a larger obedience to the laws of God "manifest in the flesh"--obedience that takes into account the moral science, the physics and the chemistry of digestion.

These and those others who have had their lives redeemed from lingering death through the simple, easy ways of Nature never suffer their enthusiasm to wane. Not to volunteer aid when unintentional suicide is going on seems nothing less than criminal.

As a means to better health the utility of the morning fast is beyond estimate. In all other modes of health culture there is a great deal of time consumed in certain exercises that are certain to be given up in time. What the busy world requires is a mode to gain and maintain the health that requires neither time nor thought--one that is really automatic.

We arise in the morning with our brain recharged by sleep, and we go at once about our business. If we take a walk or go to the gymnasium, we simply waste that much time, and we also lessen the stored-up energy by whatever of effort is called out. We can skip the dumb-bells and perform any other kind of exercise that is good for the health; and always with the certainty that we shall have more strength for the first half of the day if none is wasted in this way. As a matter of mere enjoyment, walks in fresh air are beneficial, but not as an enforced exercise for the reason of health.

For the highest possibilities for a day of human service there must be a night of sound sleep; and then one may work with muscle or with mind much longer without fatigue if no strength is wasted over untimely food in the stomach, no enforced means to develop health and strength. When one has worked long enough to become generally tired there should be a period of rest, in order to regain power to digest what shall be so eaten as to cause the brain the least waste of its powers through failure to masticate.

One need not always wait until noon to eat the first meal. Those in good health have found that they can easily go till noon before breaking the fast; but in proportion as one is weak or ailing the rule should be to stop all work as soon as fatigue becomes marked, and then rest until power to digest is restored. To eat when one is tired is to add a burden of labor to all the energies of life, and with the certainty that no wastes will be restored thereby.

For the highest efforts of genius, of art, of the simplest labors of the hands, the forenoon with empty stomach and larger measure of stored-up energy of the brain is by far the better half of the day; and, more than this, it is equally the better for the display of all the finer senses of the tastes, the finer emotions of soul life. In addition to these--and what is vastly more important--it is by far the better half of the day for the display of that energy whereby disease is cured. All this with no power lost in any special exercise for the health!

The time to stop the forenoon labor is when the need to rest has become clearly apparent; and there must be rest before eating, to restore the energy for digestion. This always determines Nature's time when the first meal shall be taken, and not the hour of the day.

This is especially important to all who are constitutionally weak or have become disabled through ailings or disease. Disappointments have come to hundreds who have given up breakfasts, because of the mistaken idea that they must wait till noon before breaking the fast, and hence had become too tired to digest; and therefore experienced a loss rather than a gain from the untimely noon meals.

The desire for morning food is a matter of habit only. Morning hunger is a disease under culture, and they who feel the most need have the most reason to fast into higher health. They who claim that their breakfasts are their best meals; that they simply "cannot do one thing" until they have eaten, are practically in line with those who must have their alcoholics before the wheels can be started.

Now it has been found by the experience of thousands that by wholly giving up the morning meal all desire for it in time disappears, which could hardly be the case if the laws of life were thereby violated; and the habit once fully eradicated is rarely resumed.

To give up suddenly the use of alcoholics or of tobacco in any of its forms is to call out loudest protests from the morbid voices that have been kept silent by those soothing powers; and yet no one would accept those loud cries as indicating an actual physiological need. The difficulties arising from giving up the morning meals--even as those from giving up the morning grog--are an exact measure of the need that they shall be given up in order that health, and not disease, shall be under culture.

I once heard a Rev. Mrs. tell a large audience of ministers that for more than a week she spent most of her forenoons in bed to endure better the headaches and other angry, protesting voices that were averse to the no-breakfast plan. She won her case, and thence on a hint of headache or other morbid symptoms was a matter of humiliation and fasting, with prayer for forgiveness and for greater moral strength against the temptations of relish.

With many people the breaking of the breakfast habit costs only less of will-power than is called out by attempts to break the alcoholic or tobacco habit; but by persistence a complete victory is certain for all, and the forenoons become a luxury of power in reserve.

Now, I must warn all that very many persons who adopt the No-breakfast Plan are disappointed, because they have become chronic in the ways of unwitting sin: they are like thin-soiled farms long-cropped without soil culture. Harvests in either case can only come by the study and practice of the laws of nutrition.

The besetting sin against all such ailing mortals, the lines of whose lives are frequently of the hardest, is that the friends all oppose cutting down the daily food from the dreadfully mistaken impression that weakness and debility from disease are the measure of the need to eat, not the measure of the inability to digest.

Scores of times I have been written to by this class of patients as to their troubles from friends in this way. Scores of times I have been consulted as to the safety of this method in daily living for the old, as if it were a tax upon the constitutional powers to stop sinning against them! As well ask whether one may get too old as to make it dangerous to cut down daily whiskey or daily labor that is clearly beyond the reasonable use of the powers.

Those who are the victims of chronic diseases and have become greatly enfeebled by overwork of body, mind, or stomach, will have to work out their salvation with most discouragingly slow progress; but not to work, not to try, is to invite the processes of disease culture.

Now, as to the time when that first meal of the day shall be taken. Since the best meal of the day in all America with the great majority of the people is at noon, this time may well be selected as the most fitting. Since the man of muscle loses no time in taking his breakfast, he should be able with good sense to rest an hour before this noon meal.

Those whose general energies give out earlier in the morning and do not care to have general meals prepared in advance of the usual hour, can put in the time in the best possible way by resting into power of relish and digestion, the evil of eating when tired being that the exhausted feeling is only increased.

Now think what forenoons may be had with no time lost over breakfasts, none in thinking about the health or in doing anything for it, and not only to have the best and strongest use of the reason, judgment, and muscles, but also to have the best possible conditions for the cure of ailings! Think, too, what it would be to the mothers of the land not to have any need to go into their kitchens until the time to prepare the noon meal arrived!

Can children while growing rapidly do without breakfasts? They certainly can without a hint of discomfort, and be all the better for it in every way.

A few months ago I spent some hours in Illinois, where the no-breakfast plan had been practised for two years. When the plan was begun there was a pale, delicate mother of four children, who was enduring a life that had no cheer. During the first year the battle was a severe one, not a little aggravated by the assurance of all sympathetic friends that resulting evil was making its mark on all the lines of expression; but health with its life and color finally came to silence the uttered disapproval.

There was a boy in the home who was subject to the severest headaches every week, and who was much wasted in his body when he began: he had become robust and wholly relieved of all his ailings. There was a plump, rosy-cheeked girl of fourteen who for a year had taken only one daily meal, and yet a better nourished body I never saw.

Now in this family the only warm, general meal, and this a plain one, was at noon. The evening meal was entirely of bread and butter taken without even a sitting at the table. What happy, healthy children they were! And the mother was in a great deal better health to do all the work of the kitchen: work, she strongly asserted, which was not nearly half of what it formerly was. For her there was a cure, a great increase of strength, and a great reduction of the most taxing of all the duties of the home-life.

If there is such a thing as an attack of disease, it cannot occur in the forenoon when there is an empty stomach and all the powers are at their best for resisting disease; and where children are fed as these are, disease, acute or chronic, is only a remote possibility.

I belong to a family of seven; the oldest is beyond seventy, the youngest beyond fifty. This No-breakfast Plan has been very closely adhered to with all for not less than twelve years, and during this time not one of us has had any acute sickness; and I am not aware that any have diseases of the chronic kind.

The accompanying illustration is that of Mrs. E. A. Quiggle, sister of the Author, after twelve years' trial of The No-breakfast Plan.

IX.

The utility of eating with thoroughness is strongly illustrated in the following cases:

Mr. Horace Fletcher, the author and traveller, took to the one-daily-meal plan to cut down his abnormal weight, having the patience to masticate all sense of taste from each mouthful before swallowing. I saw him after he had been on this plan for some months: there had been a weight loss of some forty pounds; a nasal catarrh of many years had been cured, and he strongly asserted that in every way he felt himself twenty-five years younger.

He had been living a week on baked potatoes for experimental reasons when I met him, and without experiencing any morbid sensations: a more perfect specimen of physical health I never gazed upon. To all dyspeptics who are willing to work for their health through pains and patience, his little work, Glutton or Epicure, is strongly recommended.

A dyspeptic from Vermont came to me who for ten years had eaten three hearty meals daily, none of which had ever satisfied his hunger. He was in a very low mental state when he came, and feeble in body: for fully ten years both himself and physician had held the stomach accountable for all its complainings, and with no thought of avoidable cause.

I put him on one meal a day, as there was still some power of digestion, and with the following list for the daily bill of fare: baked potatoes well buttered, bread and butter, beans dressed with butter, fish or lamb chops, and rice or oatmeal only if strongly desired; all sugar foods debarred, and no drinks except water as thirst called for it between the meals. The constipated bowels were permitted their own times for action. The mouthfuls were small and far apart--like dashes between words--not less than forty-five minutes were spent in masticating. Very soon there was a general rousement of new life in every way. His first surprise was in an unwonted sense of relish and a complete sating of hunger long before he had eaten the old-time amounts.

There was a fresh revelation to me in this, as I had not before been so impressed that by slow eating the hunger-spell is also dissipated in part by time, and hence there is much less danger of eating to excess. Hunger comes in part from habit, and it is appeased, with or without eating, with equal completeness. The hunger-habit can be trained to come at almost any fixed time.

Not long since I read of a farmer who kept his horses in apparently perfect condition on one feeding, and only at night: they had become so trained that they had no desire for food until their labors were over. At night they both ate and rested, and made good the waste of the day; they were fully nourished and rested by morning, and could labor all the forenoon without loss of energy diverted to digestion: at noon they would rest--become strong for the labors of the day.

There can be no doubt, I think, that the strongest sense of hunger at the regular eating-time could be dissipated by a fast not longer in duration than that of an ordinary meal-time.

My patient's bowels gave no hint of their locality until the eighteenth day, when they acted with little effort; on the twenty-fourth day again in a perfect way, and thereafter daily. The mind became ecstatic through perfect relief from mental and physical depression; there were no wants for other than those simple foods, and at the end of a month he left me with new views as to Nature's power of selection to meet her needs and of the vast utility of using both time and food to dissipate hunger.

The waste with most people is so small that the cost of the food, the cost of time in preparation, could be reduced to a startling fraction if the need could be actually known, and the pleasures of the palate increased by an inverse ratio. There is no redemption for women on the earth who have the care of kitchens except through simpler, smaller meals--meals so very far apart that there shall be a maximum of the hunger-sense of relish and the resulting maximum of power to convert them into tissues instinct with life.

It may be that the waste is so very trifling, especially with brain-workers, that one may be a vegetarian, fruitarian, or even an eater of pork, without positive violence to practical physiology. There is this further very practical consideration, that when Nature is so fairly dealt with that she can speak in natural tones she will call only for those foods easily available along geographical lines.

There is this to be said about fruits, that all those containing acids decompose the gastric juice, as they all contain potash salts in union with fruit acids. As soon as they reach the stomach the free hydrochloric acid of the gastric juice unites with the potash, setting the fruit acid free to irritate the stomach. There is never any desire for acid fruits through real hunger, especially those of the hyperacid kinds: they are simply taken to gratify that lower sense--relish.

The tropical fruits are without acids, and therefore are well adapted to a class of people who have only the least use for muscle and brains. Acid fruits can only be taken with apparent impunity by the young and old, who can generate gastric juice copiously. Because of the general impression that they are healthful and no tax, human stomachs are converted into cider-mills at will, regardless of between meal-times. By their ravishing flavor and apparent ease of digestion apples still play an important part in the "fall of man" from that higher estate, the Eden without its dyspepsia.

What shall we eat? The fig-leaved savage under his bread-fruit tree, the fur-clad Eskimo in his ice-hut, need not be asked: the needed food is in all due supply with little cost of muscle and less of mind--and he has no mental condition that can disturb the digestion.

The simpler waste-restoring foods have a flavor of their own that needs little reinforcement if developed by due mastication and with adequate hunger. In my own case butter duly salted seems to be my only natural appetizer aside from hunger; and yet I must own that at times new honey has a wonderful effect on the mouth-glands.

The difference between eating from hunger and mere relish, as fruits and the various sweetened foods are eaten, is a new study in dietetics, and one more important can scarcely be conceived. It can hardly be intelligently studied without taking into due account this new physiology. With rarest exceptions the need of food is estimated by the mere pleasure that comes from relish--that kind of relish that is evolved from the pies, puddings, ice creams, the last course in Sunday dinners, never taken until the limits of stomach expansion are nearly reached.

X.

Some of the external evidences of that general regeneration which comes through Nature will now be given. We will study the human face as we study the earth when the favoring conditions of Spring rouse all Nature to newness of life. The face shall be our human landscape.

I select a face in which the eyes are dull from debility, in which there is no sparkle of soul, and beneath are the dark venus-hanging clouds. The face has a dull, lifeless cast; the veins are all enlarged from debility, and cover the larger arteries as with a mourner's pall, save where there are patches as of clouds on fire, where disease of the skin enlivens the drear landscape. There are pimples large and small, some with overflowing volcanoes; there are no lines of expression: these are changed to lines of morbid anatomy. We listen, and there are no echoes of departed joys; look as we will, and we see no evidence of the existence of a soul.

The ultimate of this picture is death from unrecognized suicide; death, a slow dying to every sense that made life worth living. There is this about these deaths that go on through the months and years: they exaggerate the worst instincts of the soul as it is dragged down--down through brain-wasting largely avoidable if only understood.

The instant result of a total suspension of the use of the brain power in the digestive tract is the evolution of life: new life is sent to the remotest cell as by an electric charge. The nutrient vessels of the eye tone down in size, and there is polish, sparkle where there was only dimness; and on the face the venus clouds, black and red, begin to disappear; the toning of the veins condenses the skin, and thereby the ruddy arteries are uncovered, and a color that has life appears; the pimples, the hillocks, even have a brighter look as they slowly shrink from sight. Finally, the skin becomes of a plush-like texture, soft, condensed, and with tints that compare as the tints of flowers with the faded colors of the house-painter, or as the matchless tint and plush of the perfect peach to the spotted, colorless, wilted, degenerated representative awaiting the garbage-barrel; and the cherry lips, the cherry gums, and the whiter teeth--Nature does not match them otherwheres.

Landscape gardening upon the human face has the largest, most inspiring possibilities; and there are no eyes so dull, no faces so void of light and life, no skin degraded to a parchment, for a public display of an assorted collection of evidences of physical poverty, in which these changes to a higher life are not in some degree easily possible.

Face culture becomes of the profoundest interest when it is realized that whatever there is in eyes and lines of expression that reveals a soul in higher life, whatever there is in softness and delicacy of texture, in color that is alive with life, is only the external revelations of the higher life within. Nature is always at work over her waste places, whether about the roots in the mouth, or in the depths of the organs; and the aches, the pains of the living, and the agonies of the dying are only evidences of the earnestness and persistence of her efforts to right all her wrongs.

In what ways are drugs available in this kind of landscape culture; how sent through the crystalline structures of the eye with clearing effect; how to polish the retina and the surfaces to a sparkle? What drugs for such culture? And yet the materia medica needs a hoist to place it on the shelf. These external changes that become clearly apparent to even dull eyes are the changes that also go on in the very depths of diseased structure, in all the special senses, in all those higher instincts and tastes that make man the best for self, for home, State and Nation--the image of his Creator. Is this high estate ever reached through dosage?

Let this matter be again considered. In the days of the lancet, roots and herbs, of bleedings and sweatings, of fevers without water for parched tongues, throats, and stomachs, Nature had no part in the cure of disease in the professional or lay mind, except in rare instances in which there were those specially gifted with insight as well as eyesight.

Now such barbarism was inflicted with intense force of conviction, and it was patiently endured with the largest faith. When a mere child I was a witness of the bleeding treatment upon my mother of saintly memory, and my child hands carried into the back yard nearly a quart of blood drawn for a bilious attack that lasted but a few days.

There is this to be taken into account in the dose treatment of diseases--that most cases recover regardless of the time of treatment, even whether it is the most crucifying or whether there is no dosing. Therefore, the good effect of dosing is at best a matter of hazy inference, where real evidence is not possible. The lack of uniformity in the character and times of doses for similar diseases is a burlesque on science. What would a text-book on chemistry be worth with nothing more in the way of demonstrative evidence than we find in our materia medica in the summing up of the "medical properties" of drugs.

In modern times homoeopathy has come in as a protest against the drawing of blood and the administration of drugs that corrode. For a form of skin disease sulphur has been given by the teaspoonful by my brethren of the "regular" school; with equal faith, my brethren of the homoeopathic school will give the fraction of a grain whose denominator will cross an ordinary page: at which extreme is the science of dosage, if any; or where between? I can hardly resist the conclusion that faith in dosage is, by as much, inability for the deduction of science.

"I know whereof I believe," is the language of Science. "I believe," is the language of credulity--with all the ways back to cause too hazy for the perception of even the assuring guide-boards. Said that prince of American humorists, Artemus Ward, "I have known a man who drank one drink of whiskey every day, and yet lived to be one hundred years old; but do not believe, therefore, that by taking two drinks a day you will live to be two hundred years old." "I have known a man who had not a single tooth, and yet he could play a bass drum better than any man I ever knew;" but do not infer that the pulling of sound teeth will aid in bringing out all the possibilities of harmony, melody, and delicacy of tone of this particular instrument of song without words. I have seen a man seemingly in perfect health at one hundred years old who had eaten three meals a day; but may I infer that on four meals a day he would have lived to be one hundred and thirty-three and a third years old? A hundred times I have been told by physicians that they have had the best results from certain drugs; but in not one instance was any reason for their faith advanced.

If I am to be governed by impressions as to the utility of what I may do for the sick, what is more impressive than to draw blood as they of old did, with recovery in most cases? Have we reduced the mortality of disease by a change in dosage? If so, how much, apart from the better sanitary conditions of living and from those involved in the care of the sick?

I can easily see or believe there is utility in clearing the digestive tract at an early date in the case of severe sickness; I know that stomach and bowels are as machines run by brain power; but beyond this the materia medica is summed up in this way, "I dose my sick: they get well: therefore my treatment is successful; or if they die, it is the providence of God"--and with no thought that it may have been the providence of bad treatment.

Men and brethren of the medical profession, you believe me a heretic in all my professional modes, and only endure me because I do not carry violent hands; but you would bar the sick-room from the bleeder of old. I may attack the lancet, the herbs, the ground-roots, whose doses were only as kindling-wood and sawdust a little more refined, and you will say "Amen" with emphasis. "But we, we live in a more enlightened age: our doses are more refined"--yes, but you administer them with the same force of conviction as to their utility in the cure of disease, and with little thought as to just why they are given and how they act.

It is my present conception that feeding the sick as now very generally practised will be held, in a more enlightened age, as we now hold the lancet of a darker age--a twin relic of barbarism; and there will be only wonder that attempts were ever made to convert the lower bowel into a temporary stomach thirty feet away.

How discriminating this deputy stomach that it selects the predigested food-ration from its unutterable lower bowel involvements; sending it pure and undefiled as ready-made flesh into the blood, only requiring it to be placed as bricks to a wall. Fortunately, these lower stomachs are not subject to nausea no matter how capable of otherwise rebelling, as they so often do.

Predigested foods! If they nourish the sick, why not feed the well; why not abolish our kitchens at an immense saving in the time, expense, and worry of cooking, and live on them at an immense saving of the tax of digestion and the indigestive processes? Brethren of the medical profession, make haste to let the world know when you have found a case in which you have made use of the lower bowel so to nourish the sick body that it did not waste while the cure was going on.

THE FASTING-CURE.

XI.

NOTES AND PRESS COMMENTS ON VOLUNTARY FASTS.

The first voluntary protracted fast for the cure of chronic ailing to reach the public prints as a matter of interesting news occurred in the case of Mr. C. C. H. Cowan, of Warrensburg, Ill., early in 1899. He had been on the two-meal plan for a time, and wishing for something more radical wrote to me as to his entering upon a fast. I probably wrote him as I now find it necessary to write all who feel that fasts are necessary and cannot have my personal care, "Go on a fast and stick to it until hunger comes or until your friends begin to suffer the pangs of sympathetic starvation; then compromise with the sin of ignorance by eating the least that will bring peace to their troubled souls."

The results were summed up by the Morning-Herald Dispatch, Decatur, Ill., April 16, 1899:

"A few years ago Dr. Tanner, in New York City, fasted for forty days and forty nights, and all the world wondered. Up to that time the feat was considered impossible. From day to day the papers told of his actions and his condition, and the entire people became deeply interested in the performance. Medical men and scientists became interested in the performance, and the laity watched the faster through curiosity. Tanner's accomplishment was considered marvellous by the medical profession and laymen alike, but Dr. Tanner has long since been a back number, and his performance is not now regarded as remarkable, although there are not many persons who would care to attempt the fast. Tanner was simply trying to prove that the thing could be done. He did it, and within a year the man who held the attention of the people of the country for forty days was a visitor to this city. What Tanner did has been more than accomplished by a Macon County man, but he went about his undertaking quietly, and the fact that he was fasting was known to only a few of his friends. The man is C. C. H. Cowan, of Warrensburg, and for forty-two days and nights he abstained from the use of food in solid or liquid form. He began his fast on March 2 and broke it on the evening of April 13 at supper-time. With the exception of the loss of thirty pounds of flesh, which materially changed his personal appearance, Mr. Cowan shows no ill-effects of his undertaking. When he began he weighed one hundred and sixty-five pounds, and when he quit he weighed one hundred and thirty-five pounds.

Before his fast he was inclined to be fleshy, and now, while still in fairly good flesh, his clothing manifests a desire not to hold close communion with his body. Mr. Cowan was in the city Saturday, and some of his friends did not know him. He related his experience to some of them, but he did this cautiously, and with the oft-expressed hope that the papers would not devote any attention to the affair, because he was not seeking and did not want notoriety. At different times during his fast the Herald-Dispatch has referred to the fact in short items. Cowan is a disciple of a Dr. Dewey, living at Meadville, Pa., who is an advocate of fasting as a means of curing many of the ills to which the body is heir. Dr. Dewey has many pamphlets touching the subject, and has also written some books for his belief, and his reasons have been made so plausible that a number of persons have coincided with him. Cowan says the efficacy of the treatment has been established in many instances, a fact that he can prove by ample testimony. During his long abstinence from food he had numerous letters and telegrams from Dr. Dewey, encouraging him in the undertaking. When asked why he had fasted, Cowan explained that for years he had suffered from chronic nasal and throat catarrh which would not yield to medical treatment. His appetite was splendid, and he ate many things that he really did not want. He read Dr. Dewey's ideas, and became convinced that his system needed general overhauling, and that this could be accomplished through faithful adherence to the theory of Dr. Dewey. One of these theories is to the effect that fasting rests the brain, which is ofttimes overworked as a result of heavy feeding. It is also supposed that the body throws off old mucous membrane of the stomach and bowels, and that these are immediately supplanted by new lining. Believing that he could get rid of his catarrhal trouble and get the new lining referred to, Cowan decided to fast, and without noise about the matter he commenced, and up to Thursday evening he did not allow a bite of food to pass his lips. The only thing that he took was water. Of this he did not drink much, and he claims that he suffered no pain or pangs of hunger. Looking at the matter now, it does not seem to have been much of an accomplishment. After he once got started he said it was an easy matter to carry out his plan except for the worry of his family and some of his friends. They thought that he was losing his mind and tried to induce him to relinquish his idea, but he took some of them under his wing and reasoned with them on the beauties of the treatment, expounded the strong points, gave them reasons, showed them testimony of others, and kept on fasting. When he began he had no idea that he would continue for forty days; but as he progressed he had no desire for food, and therefore did not desist. Thursday evening he began to feel hungry, and that night he ate a reasonably good supper. The return of hunger, according to his theories, was the signal of the return of health. He feels confident that his stomach has been relined, and for the present he knows that his catarrh has left him. He is a firm believer in the new method of curing bodily ailments, and says that during his fast he was able to be around the village of Warrensburg every day, and was able to perform his duties. His abstinence from food apparently has not weakened his constitution. Since breaking his fast he has partaken sparingly of food. Cowan's friends are very much interested in the recital of his experience."

It so chanced that during this fast much more than his ordinary business came to him, and without the least inability to perform it. I saw him several months later, and found his physical condition seemingly perfect. He had found out that for the best working conditions a nap at noon was better than even a light luncheon, and that one meal a day taken after his business was over was the best practice. This fast was not in the right locality to excite the attention it deserved.

The second voluntary fast was destined to reach the ends of the earth through the public prints. The following appeared in the New York Press of June 6, 1899:

"Twenty-eight days without nourishment and without letting up for a moment on the daily routine of his business is the unequalled record of Milton Rathbun, a hay and grain dealer at No. 453 Fourth Avenue, and living in Mount Vernon. He is a man of wealth, has many employés, and has been in the same business in this city for thirty-nine years.

"He fasted because he wanted to reduce his weight, fearing that its gradual increase might bring on apoplexy. He succeeded in his efforts. He weighed two hundred and ten pounds when he stopped eating; when he resumed he tipped the scales at one hundred and sixty-eight pounds, a loss of forty-two pounds of flesh.

"Mr. Rathbun's description of how he felt as the days and weeks wore along and the pounds of avoirdupois slipped away one by one is interesting. The remarkable point about it is that he continued his work and kept well. He gave his account of it yesterday to a reporter for The Press. Mr. Rathbun is known by the business men for blocks around his own place of business, and they all know of his fast.

"Every day his friends would come in and talk to him about it. At first they told him he was foolish; that nobody could fast that length of time, much less continue his work without interruption. Then as the days went on and he kept up without a break they began to be frightened.

"A crowd would gather about him every night at 6.30 o'clock, when he would leave his office, for that was his hour for weighing. Some days he would lose two or three pounds from the weight of the day before; some days only one, but always something. And as the record was scored up on the book each night his friends would shake their heads and warn him to beware.

"Finally, on the fifteenth day, his friends and employ 閣 got together and made up their minds that something had to be done. They were afraid that Rathbun would die. They appointed a committee to wait on him in his office and beg him to eat something. The committee took dainties to Mr. Rathbun, told him their fears, and offered the good things to tempt him, but all to no purpose.

"It was the night of April 23 that Mr. Rathbun took his last bit of nourishment. He made no attempt to eat a large meal in preparation for his fast. He ate his regular supply just as if he had meant to continue eating on the following day. Then for twenty-eight days he absolutely abjured all food. He drank water, but that was all. Before going to bed he would take a pint of Apollinaris.

"Had he remained at his home in bed or taken perfect rest, his achievement would have been less remarkable. That is the course which always has been adopted by the professional fasters. Dr. Tanner, and the Italian, Succi, in their fasts were surrounded by attendants who allowed them scarcely to lift a hand, so that every ounce of energy might be conserved.

"Rathbun pursued a course diametrically opposite to this. He worked, and worked hard. He came down earlier to his office and went away later than usual. He made no effort to save himself. On the contrary, he seemed determined to make his task as hard as possible. On four of his fast days he spent the afternoons in a dentist's chair, at which times his nerves were tried as only dentists know how to do it.

"It was his idea to continue the fast until he began to feel hunger. After the first twenty-four hours his hunger disappeared, and he had no desire for food until the end of the fourth week, when the craving set in, and he immediately set about satisfying it in a moderate and careful manner. He consulted two physicians while the fast was going on, to see that he was suffering no injury that he could not appreciate himself. One was Dr. F. B. Carpenter, of Madison Avenue and thirty-eight Street, and the other, Dr. George J. Helmer, of Madison Avenue and Thirty-first Street. He saw Dr. Carpenter on the eighteenth and the twenty-first days, and Dr. Helmer on the twenty-fifth day. Both expressed surprise at his long fast and astonishment at his excellent condition.

"Mr. Rathbun is fifty-four years old, and five feet six inches in height. He does not look more than forty years old, and he is as active as a man of that age. He says he never felt better than when he was fasting, and that he has experienced no bad effects of any kind, while, on the other hand, he has reduced his weight to a normal limit and removed all danger of apoplexy.

"He got the idea of the fast from the new theory exploited by Dr. Edward Hooker Dewey, a practising physician of Meadville, Pa., who recommends fasting as a cure for many ailments, and advises all persons to go without breakfast and eat only two meals a day.

"'I became intensely interested in this new system,' said Mr. Rathbun yesterday, 'and I decided to put it to a practical test. Dr. Dewey had said that he had many patients fasting all the way from ten to thirty and forty days, and I concluded that if it did them so much good it would be just the thing for me. So I tried it.

"'On April 23 I ate my last meal, and from then until May 24 I had absolutely nothing to eat. I drank water, of course, for that is a matter of necessity. One cannot do without drink; but I took no nourishment. For the first twenty-four hours I was very hungry, and would have liked very much to take a square meal; but I resisted the temptation, and after the expiration of one day I had no desire to eat.

"'I had been in the habit of getting to my office about 8; now I get there at 7. I generally had left at 5.30; I now stayed until 6.30. I had been in the habit of taking an hour or an hour and a quarter for luncheon. The luncheon was now cut off, so I stayed in the office and worked. I sat there at my desk and put in a long, hard day's work, constantly writing.

"'At night I drank a bottle of Apollinaris, and went to bed at 8.30 and slept until 4 in the morning. I never enjoyed better sleep than in those four weeks. And I was in excellent condition as far as I could see in every other way. My mind was clear, my eye was sharper than usually, and all the functions were in excellent working order.

"'I had many amusing experiences. I went to a dentist on the first day. I had some work requiring several hours' labor on the part of the dentist. I said nothing to the doctor on the first day. Four or five days afterward I kept a second appointment with the dentist, and he asked me how the teeth worked which he had fixed before. I said to him: "I haven't tried them yet."

"'You can imagine the look of surprise on his face. When I told him that I was fasting, and had been since he had seen me before, he showed the greatest concern, and said he did not think I could go on with the dental work on account of the weakness of my nerves. He solicited me to go out and have just a bite of something. I refused, of course, and he continued the work. I visited him on two days after that until he had finished the work.

"'The men in my employ were greatly concerned about me, and thought I would break down. I used to weigh every night before leaving the office, and as they saw my constant wearing away they became more and more frightened, and finally appointed a committee to wait on me. The committee was headed by my manager, who begged me to eat. He brought along some fine ripe cherries to tempt me. I told him I would not eat them for one thousand dollars, for I was interested thoroughly in the fast by that time and would not have stopped.

"'After that they made no more attempts to stop the fast; but my friends all shook their heads, and said that when I started in to eat again I would find I was without a proper stomach.

"'On the twenty-eighth day the hunger began to come on again, and I began to eat under the advice of Dr. Carpenter. On the twenty-ninth day I drank a little bouillon, and afterward from day to day increased the amount of food to the normal. I suffered no inconvenience.'

"Mr. Rathbun says he is a firm believer in the no-breakfast system of hygiene advocated by Dr. Dewey, and that neither himself, his wife, nor any of the servants in his house eat breakfast, and as a result all are remarkably well. His two sons, one of whom was graduated at Harvard in 1896, and a second, who is still at Harvard, practise the no-breakfast system.

"Just before beginning his fast Mr. Rathbun ordered a suit of clothes at his tailor's. He did not go for it until the end of his long fast. Being something of a practical joker, besides a man of great nerve, he walked into the tailor-shop and let the tailor try his new suit on to see if it was all right.

"When he slipped on the coat the tailor stood aghast. There was apparently the same man he had measured twenty-eight days previously standing before him in perfect health, but as to dimensions not at all the same man.

"'It doesn't fit any part of you,' said the tailor, after the suit had been tried on. In the tailor's book Rathbun's measurement was entered: 'Forty-three inches around the waist and forty-two around the chest.' When he went for his suit his measurements were thirty-eight around the waist and thirty-eight around the chest.

"Dr. Dewey's theory, which led Rathbun to make his long fast, is that the brain is the centre of every mind and muscle energy, a sort of self-charging dynamo, with the heart, lungs, and all the other parts only as so many machines to be run by it; that the brain has the power of feeding itself on the less important parts of the body without loss of its own structure, and that as the operation of digestion is a tax on the brain, a long period of fasting gives the brain a rest, by which means the brain is able to build itself up, which means the upbuilding of the whole body.

"In this way, it is asserted, the alcohol habit is cured and other diseases eradicated.

"Dr. F. B. Carpenter said yesterday to a reporter for The Press that he had not recommended Mr. Rathbun to take the fast, but had advised him while it was going on and after it was over. The doctor said he was inclined to believe there might be something in the no-breakfast system, as a great many persons eat and drink altogether too much.

"Dr. Helmer said he had examined Rathbun on the twenty-fifth day, and had found him in surprisingly good condition."

Mr. Rathbun had been on the no-breakfast plan for several years, and he was one of the first to write me after my book came out. It was not without reason he feared apoplexy, for Ex-Gov. Flower, an over-weighted man, had gone down to instant death though seemingly in perfect health and in the prime of business energy and mental capacity. During his fast my only trouble with him was in his drinking so much water without thirst, thus greatly and needlessly adding to the work of the kidneys.

Mr. Rathbun was so disappointed over the skepticism of New York physicians as to the reliability of the fast that he determined to undergo a longer one under such surveillance as would enforce conviction. He was mainly actuated, however, to go through the ordeal in the interests of science.

Again I had trouble with him on the water question, wishing him to drink only as thirst incited. He was differently advised by an eminent Boston physician, who, taking a great interest in the case, wrote him that he should have great care to drink certain definite amounts for the necessary fluidity of the blood. I had to respond that thirst would duly indicate this need; that in my cases of protracted fasts from acute sicknesses not one had been advised to take even a teaspoonful of water for such reasons; that at the closing days before recovery of such cases there was only the least desire for water, and this with no indication of need from the blood. Mr. Rathbun did not escape some trouble from overworked kidneys, and he became convinced that my theory and practice were more in line with physiology.

This fast was made a matter of daily record by the leading New York journals, and he became such a subject of general interest that in addition to his ordinary business he was greatly overtaxed, and was compelled to give up the fast on the thirty-fifth day, in part from the exhaustion of over-excitement.

This case was summed up as follows by the New York Press, February 27, 1900:

"Milton Rathbun has ended his long fast.

"After thirty-five days, in which solid food or any liquid other than water was a stranger to his palate, he became extremely hungry on Sunday night. At first he resisted the longing to eat and tried to sleep it off. But he awoke in a few hours hungrier than ever, and then he decided he had fasted as long as was good for him.

"He ate a modest, light meal and went back to bed, only to awake still hungry. Then he ate an orange, and was asleep again in a jiffy. A bowl of milk and cream and crackers sufficed for his breakfast, and at noon yesterday he enjoyed his first hearty meal.

"As he walked around the parlor of his home in Mount Vernon, lighter by forty-three pounds than he was on January 21, this man of fifty-five years and iron will said:

"'I feel like a boy again. I think I could vault over a six-foot fence.'

"Mrs. Rathbun herself knows what it is to fast. For five years such a thing as breakfast has been an unknown quantity in her house, save when guests were present or for the servants. To this abstinence Mrs. Rathbun attributes the curing of catarrh, from which she had suffered previously. And as she and her husband do, so do their two sons.

"After the first few days of abstinence he had felt no desire to eat until Sunday evening. Then he became hungry--ravenously so. His first fast of a year ago--it was twenty-eight days then--had taught him that sleep took away the longing for food, and, too, he had said he would make his fast last forty days this time. So he went to bed and to sleep.

"But he awoke at 11 o'clock; he was hungrier than ever, and he decided not to resist his inclination for food. Calling his wife he asked her for an orange, and ate it; then he took another. His next demand was for oysters, and a dozen large, juicy ones disappeared rapidly, to the accompaniment of five soda crackers. Then he drank about two-thirds of a cup of beef-tea, and some Oolong tea. His appetite was not sated by any means, but he knew the danger of overloading his stomach, so he stopped.

"He soon was slumbering again, but he was wide awake at 2 o'clock in the morning. And his hunger was with him still. He ate an orange to appease the craving, and again sought his pillow. He slept again until 6 o'clock, and then, breaking some crackers in a bowl of milk and cream, he ate again.

"At noon a meal was served to the still hungry man. He began with a little clam-broth; then came half a dozen steamed clams, followed by a small portion of mock-turtle soup. Of a squab he ate one-half, and with it some canned pease and fried potatoes; while for dessert he had a little lemon ice.

"'That was good,' he exclaimed, as he finished. The remark was unnecessary; the relish with which he had eaten was convincing testimony of his enjoyment. Asked why he had decided not to fast for the full forty days, he said:

"'I ate just because I was hungry.'

"Asked how the weather affected him, he said:

"'When I began there was a spell of cold weather, and I found it rather hard to keep warm at night. But it soon passed away, and I made it a point to wear the same underclothing and outer garments as usual. Oh, yes; I did wear a different pair of trousers. I had them made five years ago, but they were so tight around the waist I could never wear them. They are as loose as can be now, however.'

"'From a scientific standpoint,' said Professor R. Ogden Doremus yesterday, 'it is the most interesting and valuable experiment I have known. Mr. Rathbun is a man of great nerve force. The very fact that he attended to his business was what saved him, in keeping his mind away from the thought of food. He could not have done it had he been on exhibition or if he had remained at home. If he had been at sea, in an open boat, he could not have lasted more than ten days. He would have had nothing to think of but his hunger.'

"Dr. George J. Helmer, who has given no little attention to Mr. Rathbun, said:

"'I have examined him several times; I did so when his thirty days were up. Well, it was remarkable. It's a wonderful exhibition, that will attract the attention of the medical world. His heart is as clear as a bell and his kidneys are perfect. He is in absolutely rugged health. His temperature was normal, his eye clear, and to-day, upon examination, any insurance company would rate him as an A1 risk.'

"Following is from the diary kept during his fast, and furnished by Milton Rathbun to The Press:

"First Day, Jan. 22, 8.45 A. M.--Weight, 207 pounds; height, 5 ft. 6-1/2 inches; chest measure, 43-1/2 inches; waist measure, 43-1/2 inches; hip measure, 46-1/2 inches; calf measure, 17 inches; biceps measure, 14 inches; forearm, 12 inches. 3 P. M., feels well, but hungry. In the evening felt well, not being hungry or thirsty. Have taken no water.

"Tuesday, Jan. 23.--Slept well until 6 A. M. Rested a while, then took sponge bath and rubdown. At 8.45 weighed 200 pounds. Feel good, but a little weak. 12 o'clock M., no appetite and feverish. 4 P. M., weighed 199 pounds; went home; drank one pint of water during the evening.

"Wednesday, Jan. 24.--Slept well for nine hours. Got up at 6 A. M., drank one glass of water and took train to the city. 8.30 A. M., weighed 198-1/2 pounds; only half pound lost, which shows how greedily the tissues absorb moisture and add to weight. 12 o'clock M., have no appetite nor thirst, and no fever. Retired at 9 o'clock, feeling comfortable but a little feverish.

"Thursday, Jan. 25.--After having slept seven and one-half hours took a sponge bath and brisk rubdown. Came to the city, and at 8.25 A. M. weighed 195 pounds. Feeling good, with no fever nor appetite. 4.45 P. M., weighed 193 pounds. At home during the evening drank two and one-half glasses of water.

"Friday, Jan. 26.--Slept eight hours. No appetite and feeling stronger. Examined by Professor Doremus and Dr. Carpenter. Retired at 9 o'clock, feeling first class.

"Saturday, Jan. 27.--Came to the city on the 7.45 A. M. train. Weighed 191 pounds. Feeling good. No fever and no appetite.

"Sunday, Jan. 28.--Drank one glass of water when I got up. During the day and evening drank three more glasses of water. Retired feeling first class.

"Monday, Jan. 29.--Slept eight hours last night, and came to the city on the 7.45 A. M. train. At 8.25 weighed 189 pounds. 4 P. M., was examined by Dr. F. B. Carpenter, who found the temperature 98-1/2?F., pulse regular, tongue clean. Measurements were: waist, 41 inches; chest, 41 inches; hip, 45 inches; calf, 16 inches; biceps, 13-1/2 inches; forearm, 11-1/2 inches. 5.15 P. M., weighed 188 pounds.

"Tuesday, Jan. 30.--Slept eight hours; weighed 188 pounds, same as the night before; feeling good. 5.30 P. M., weighed 185-1/2 pounds.

"Wednesday, Jan. 31.--Slept 7-1/2 hours, drank one and one-half glasses of water; weighed at 8.25 A. M. 187 pounds; Dr. Carpenter found temperature 98?F., and pulse 88; Professor Doremus called a little later; weighed 184-1/2 pounds.

"Thursday, Feb. 1.--Rested quietly when not asleep; drank only one and three-quarters glasses of water all day; weighed 184 pounds; retired feeling good.

"Friday, Feb. 2.--Not feeling any hunger; was examined by F. B. Carpenter; temperature, 98?F.; pulse, 84; weighed 183 pounds; retired feeling well, but tired.

"Saturday, Feb. 3.--Somewhat wakeful during the night. 5.45 P. M., weighed 182 pounds.

"Sunday, Feb. 4.--Read all day and felt well.

"Monday, Feb. 5.--2 P. M., temperature, 98.4?F.; pulse, 82; tongue clean. Measurements were: waist, 41 inches; chest, 41 inches; hip, 43 inches; calf, 14-1/2 inches; biceps, 13-1/2 inches; forearm, 11-1/2 inches; went to bed feeling a trifle feverish.

"Tuesday, Feb. 6.--Wakeful during the night. 11 A. M., had my eyes examined by Dr. L. H. Matthez, oculist, and found a marked improvement in my sight over same tests of two months previous, being 7 degrees stronger; felt a little weak, but no fever or appetite; weighed 180 pounds; feeling somewhat exhausted from the day's labor and in entertaining guests.

"Wednesday, Feb. 7.--Slept about seven hours during the night; when I awoke felt rested; temperature, 98.2?F.; pulse, 80; have felt well all day; went to bed at 9.30; some fever.

"Thursday, Feb. 8.--Woke up two or three times during the night. Drank water during the night and first thing this morning when I got up. Came to the city, and at 9 o'clock weighed 182 pounds, showing a gain of two pounds over last night. Not feeling so well owing to the amount of water I drank last night, which was induced by feverishness.

"Friday, Feb. 9.--Feeling first rate. At 8.25 A. M. weighed 180 pounds. Heart action normal. No enlargement of the spleen or liver.

"Saturday, Feb. 10.--Lost nothing in weight during the day and have felt well all the while.

"Sunday, Feb. 11.--Passed the day in reading and drank frequently of water.

"Monday, Feb. 12.--This being a holiday, did not go to the city. Passed the day in entertaining callers. Have not felt quite so well owing to a slight cold settling in my left kidney.

"Tuesday, Feb. 13.--Measurements: waist, 38-1/2 inches; chest, 40 inches; hip, 43 inches; calf, 14-1/2 inches; biceps, 12-1/2 inches; forearm, 11 inches; weight, 177-1/2 pounds.

"Wednesday, Feb. 14.--I attribute the cause of loss of sleep to a hard day's work and in reading too long last evening.

"Thursday, Feb. 15.--Somewhat wakeful during the night. Retired at 7.30 o'clock, after a hard day's work.

"Friday, Feb. 16.--3.30 P. M., temperature, 98.5?F.; pulse, 74; tongue clean; weighed 172-1/2 pounds. During the evening drank one cup of hot water.

"Saturday, Feb. 17.--After a restful night felt well all day.

"Sunday, Feb. 18.--Retired at 9 o'clock and have rested a good deal during the day.

"Monday, Feb. 19.--Weighed 169-1/2 pounds, and retired feeling well.

"Tuesday, Feb. 20.--Weighed 168-1/2 pounds; was examined by Dr. Helmer, who found me in excellent condition; 4.30 P. M., weighed 169-1/2 pounds, a gain of one pound during the day, on account of drinking a little more water than usual.

"Wednesday, Feb. 21.--Temperature, 98.5?F.; pulse, 69; 4 P. M., weighed 168-1/2 pounds; have not felt quite so well during the day.

"Thursday, Feb. 22.--Occupied the day--holiday--in reading and reclining, and went to bed feeling pretty well.

"Friday, Feb. 23.--At 8.30 A. M. weighed 166 pounds; 3.30 P. M., temperature, 99?F.; pulse, 98; lung expansion, 2-3/4 inches; went home and to bed, feeling considerably exhausted owing to a hard day's work and too many callers.

"Saturday, Feb. 24.--Did not rest very well from overtaxing the brain yesterday. Do not feel quite so well this morning owing to that fact and from drinking too much water during the past twenty-four hours. At 8.25 A. M. weighed 166 pounds; went home not feeling well to-day on account of some stomach disturbance, which probably comes from drinking too much water; did not drink any water during the evening; feeling quite tired at bedtime.

"Sunday, Feb. 25.--Slept nine hours and rested well, and did not drink any water during the night. Kept quiet all day, lying down most of the time, and felt the coming of hunger about 6 o'clock.

12 o'clock noon, pulse regular; tongue clean; temperature, 98; weighed 164 pounds. Measurements were: waist, 36-1/2 inches; chest, 38 inches; hip, 40-1/2 inches; calf, 14 inches; biceps, 11 inches; forearm, 10 inches.

Was in bed at 8 o'clock, still feeling hungry, and after a short sleep woke up at 11 o'clock with a sharp appetite, and ate a dozen raw oysters, two oranges, two-thirds cup of beef-tea, five crackers, and part of a cup of Oolong tea.

I insert a photograph of Mr. Rathbun taken shortly after his second fast. There had been five years' trial of the No-Breakfast Plan before these fasting demonstrations."

One of the hardest things on earth as a mental operation is to be fair to the opposition. Now lest I have beguiled my readers overmuch by the force of my convictions even to the point of danger, I will give an estimate of the danger of fasting by one of the most eminent physicians of New York City, Dr. George F. Shrady. I quote from an interview reported in the New York Sun:

"The strange case of Milton Rathbun, of Mt. Vernon, who, to reduce his flesh and generally tone up his system, is said to have gone without food of any sort for thirty-six days, still continues to be the subject of more or less discussion among the medical men of the city. Dr. George F. Shrady, in speaking last evening of Mr. Rathbun's remarkable exploit, said:

"'There are three things to say about it. In the first place, the fact, if it be a fact, as it seems to be, is astonishing; secondly, it was very foolish; and thirdly, it would be a very unfortunate and dangerous thing to popularize such experiments. Now as to whether the gentleman in question actually did go thirty-six days without taking nourishment of any sort is a matter I will not discuss. If he were a professional faster, I would hardly hesitate to say his claim was fraudulent, for I am fully convinced that all the professional fasters are frauds. They are simply adept sleight-of-hand men. They work out some adroit trick by which they may get nourishment into their systems in spite of the always more or less negligent or suspicious watchers, and then advertise for a forty days' or sixty days' 'fast.'

* * * * *

"'Now, mind you, I do not say this Mt. Vernon case is anything of this sort. I only say that if it is true it is most astounding. It is in flat contradiction of all the authorities on the subject of a human being's ability to do without food. The extreme limit of all well-authenticated cases of total abstinence from nourishment is from nine to ten days. Imprisoned miners have been known to go that time and survive.

* * * * *

"'But at all events it was a very foolish thing for Mr. Rathbun to do. About that there can be no manner of doubt. What will be the future effect upon him--upon his heart action, upon his impoverished blood, upon his nervous system, upon his organs of nutrition, necessarily paralyzed for days? These are grave questions, the answers to which may be unpleasant to Mr. Rathbun as they reveal themselves to him in the future. You cannot fly in the face of Nature and ignore all her laws in that way with impunity. She exacts her penalties and there is no court of appeals in her realm.

"'When I say that the extreme limits of abstinence from nourishment in clearly authenticated cases is from nine to ten days, you must not get the impression that all persons can last that long.

* * * * *

"'It is a question of environment, of mental condition--whether buoyed by hope or stimulated by ambition to do a great feat--and above all, of course, of the physical condition of the faster. Without food the body absorbs its own tissues. Mr. Rathbun, I am told, was a very heavy man with a superabundance of tissue. Naturally he could go longer without nourishment than a weak, attenuated, thin-blooded man.

* * * * *

"'Yet Mr. Rathbun was exercising daily and about his usual avocations, and he abstained from food for thirty-six days! Well, it's remarkable!

* * * * *

"'But I sincerely hope Mr. Rathbun will have no imitators. It would be a very unfortunate thing, fraught with grave possibilities, if the newspaper accounts of his reduction in weight and general improvement in health were to move others to follow his example. Many persons would be injured for life, physically wrecked, and perhaps actually killed if they conscientiously did the fifth part of what he is said to have done.

* * * * *

"'And right here it may be said that there is a great deal of exaggeration in the sweeping statements made about people eating too much. If a man sleeps well, goes about his business in a cheerful frame of mind, and does not get what is called "out-of-sorts," he may be pretty sure he is not eating too much, even though he eat a good deal. My observation is that the average man who works and gets a proper amount of exercise does not eat too much. If you want to get work done by the engine, you have got to stoke up the furnace. If a man wants to keep his vital energies up to par he has got to put in the fuel--that is, the food.

"'Of course, there are those who lead sedentary lives who get too much absorbed in the pleasures of the table and overfeed. There are a sufficient number of these, to be sure, but I think they are the exception. But it will be a sad mistake if even they seek a road to health by Mr. Rathbun's starvation methods.'"

The doctor is astonished, and so am I that he is astonished. This would seem to imply that he has never had cases of acute sickness in which the amount of food taken during many days or even weeks was too small to play any part as a life-prolonging factor.

"It was a foolish, even dangerous experiment." How foolish or dangerous? What vital organs suffered? Was there evidence of a loss of anything but fat? What organs were "necessarily paralyzed" during the fast? Evidently not the brain, else longer days of labor would not have been possible; and the grave future possibilities in heart action, impoverished blood, nervous system, upon organs of nutrition "necessarily paralyzed" for days; and the extreme limit of nine or ten days before death from starvation; and that without food the body lives on its own tissues!

One can easily see that the earnest doctor is full of strong impressions that have little of the flavor of science: truth that is not self-evident should have the instant logic in easy reach. I may here say that my hygienic scheme has from the first been subject to similar attacks by physicians from the standpoint of impressions, but no physician has ventured into print against it after becoming aware of its physiologic basis.

I am happy to assure all readers that in all the involuntary fasts of my cases of acute sickness or in the voluntary fasts in chronic disease, has there been any other than improved general health as the result. Notably was this the case in a man who fasted ten years ago for forty days for an ulcer of the stomach, and who had been troubled with indigestion for more than forty years. He had become nearly a mental and physical wreck when he took to his bed with an abolished appetite. There have since been some ten years of nearly perfect health, and now in his seventy-seventh year he is the youngest-looking man for his age I have ever seen. He walks the streets with the gait of a youth of twenty. To do without food without hunger does not tax any vital power, as Dr. Shrady may yet become aware.

XII.

The next fast to have a brief notoriety as the "most remarkable on record" occurred in Philadelphia, the medical center of America, and beneath the very shadow of its great medical schools; in Philadelphia, a city that surpasses all other cities for the wisest conservatism, for all-around level-headedness. Its journals are rarely equalled for their clean, winnowed columns; there is no "yellow" journalism in that great, fair city, known as the "Quaker City."

Miss Estella Kuenzel, a lady of twenty-two years, of acutest, finest sensibilities, born to live in June and not in March, lost her mental health to a degree that death became the final object of desire.

She had a friend in a bright young man of the name of Henry Ritter, chemist and photographer at the Drexel Institute, a born scientist, and who possesses the very genius of the pains and persistence of science. Well versed in the science of the morning fast, he believed that a fast which would merely end with hunger would result in all-around improvement. A fast was instituted which he thought would not last more than a few days, but went on until the days merged into weeks: it went on because only general improvement attended it.

I first heard of it in a letter written by him on the thirty-eighth day of the fast, during which there had been a walk of seven miles. On the forty-second day of the fast I had a brief letter from Miss K., in which every line was radiant with cheer.

At the Asylum five feedings per day were ordered, and at first were rejected; but finally she accepted them as a means to end her unhappy life; took them in bed, and in the last weeks seemed to be fleshing up, as there was a gain of seventeen pounds above the normal, of water--she had become dropsical. The last professional expert in her case advised a half-gallon of milk daily in addition to the three regular meals--making a five-meal plan.

To carry out an unopposed fast it was necessary to take her to a home where the parents would be ignorant of this radical means to a cure.

The following is from Mr. Ritter's letters:

"I had made my views known to the parents and daughter when the case commenced, and after the failure of these methods they decided to let me have charge of the case, which was on Sept. 30, 1899. I at once requested them to send her to the house of some friends to whom I made my views known. We then discharged the nurse who had gone with her. With doctor and nurse gone there was free room for Nature's victory (the young lady being as deeply interested as any). We put her upon the rest, which was the only needed sign since her first signs of breakdown appeared Oct. 2, at the supper table, being the last meal she has taken up to to-day, Nov. 9, this being, as you will see, the thirty-eighth day of her fast, with cheerfulness and strength holding full sway. I put her to bed on the first day, to which she kept, with an occasional day in the rocker, until the eleventh day, when she took a walk of about one mile. Then she rested indoors until the twentieth day, when we went to church, walking a little over two miles, with no fatigue or tired feelings. I forgot to mention that we had been out driving in the bracing air for over three hours in the afternoon. On the twenty-first and twenty-second days, indoors, walking and working around the house, reading, etc. On the twenty-third day walked through the country for three miles, stopping at friends to enlighten them upon 'Nature's Laws;' twenty-fourth day, eight miles, no fatigue; twenty-fifth day, between seven and eight miles, no fatigue; twenty-sixth day, walked one and a half hours; twenty-ninth day, rainy, no walks; thirtieth day, walked in the evening for two and a half hours; thirty-first day, walked seven miles, no fatigue; thirty-second day, rainy, no walks; thirty-third day, went to the Exposition, walked all day from 2 P. M. until 11.30 P. M. (with rest while at the performance we attended of not over one and a quarter hours), this being the only resting, possibly two hours, during the whole time.

"Weight taken at the start, one hundred and forty pounds; at the Exposition one hundred and twenty-five and three-quarters pounds; no sense of tired feeling, but hunger started to assert itself for a period of about three hours, after which it passed over.

"On the thirty-fourth day went driving; thirty-fifth day, walked one mile, then went to the asylum to show the results. The physicians in charge were simply astounded, and would hardly believe it possible for one to be so active while taking no food. I believe we have done quite a little good there, as they have expressed the desire to try the same on others. They examined the tongue and took the pulse, finding both in good, normal state; in the evening walked another mile, visiting the other doctors whom her parents called in. On the thirty-sixth day walked one and a half miles; thirty-seventh day, walked seven miles, hunger sensation becoming decided.

"I have given you a sketch of this case because it seems to me an unusual one owing to the great activity."

"November 18, 1899.

"Miss Kuenzel's hunger arrived as per Nature's demand on the forty-fifth day at noon. One poached egg and two slices of toast (whole wheat). There was an intense relish for her simple fare, but not the least sign or desire for haste in eating. She was amply satisfied for the day, and relished the same bill of fare and quantity for the forty-sixth day, with a very slight luncheon in the evening. We had been to the Exposition the night of the forty-fourth day, when the tongue again started cleaning and a most distinct craving for food presented itself. It persisted on retiring, and also on the next morning, when she felt that Nature again was ready for her wonderful chemistry of digestion. I had her weight taken after her first meal, which revealed a loss of twenty pounds. We called to see the professor under whom she was last placed, and he was surprised with the clearness of her mental condition and good general appearance, though he observed she had gotten a trifle thinner, but which he had also in view to accomplish upon a five-meal plan per day. He tried his best to confuse and trouble her with questions, etc., but found her too intensely awake, and she won the victory by cornering him in his own set traps. We received his congratulations and were made to promise to call again. I have now been with her to seven physicians who were interested, and have shown them Nature's own unhampered work.

"Miss Kuenzel has now an intense desire to help others. You are at liberty to make use of Nature's work in her case for the benefit of others, and I shall be only too glad to give you any desired information that may be of use. The good work you have started will, I am sure, never end; and it will prove a pleasure to me indeed to work with added interest for the benefit of those in need of the same in the future."

The forty-fourth day of the fast was the busiest of all with her. She arose at 8.30 A. M. to attend to her affairs until the late afternoon, when she and her friend met a sister, by appointment from her home, at the Exposition. Several hours were spent there, and when they took the street car for return the only vacant seat was accepted by the sister, because she was tired, and not knowing that there were forty-four days without food with her sister, who was not tired. A striking feature of these daily walks was that they did not cause marked fatigue. Miss Kuenzel retired near midnight without unusual fatigue, and so ended the forty-fourth day of the fast.

I quote from the Chester County Times of Feb. 12, 1899:

"'Conclusive evidence is being multiplied as to the wonderful power of fasting in the restoration of health, but it is only more recently that its power in the case of insanity is even yet more wonderful. A recent case is as near home as the city of Philadelphia, and those interested are very willing that others may know of it, so that its usefulness may be extended and its value appreciated. The discovery was made by Dr. E. H. Dewey, of Meadville, Pa., and tidings of the good work are being spread by Charles C. Haskell & Son, of Norwich, Conn. The editor of this paper knows somewhat the value of the discovery by an experience of several years. We give a letter from the lady who was cured.

"'PHILADELPHIA, PA., Dec. 12, 1899.

"'My Dear Mr. Haskell:

"'I have received your letter of the 9th inst., and at last find time to fulfil the request for a statement. In regard to my wonderful cure through "The New Gospel of Health," I would state that the second week after Christmas, 1898, I first had a paralyzing effect which affected the right side of face, body, and limbs, also tongue, which nearly prevented my speaking. This passed over and I again began working at my position as milliner in a large establishment, and after a short while became so dizzy and confused that I was compelled to ask my friends to direct me home. (This was around Easter, 1899.) I was then taken to a doctor, who at once requested me to stop working, and to take a complete rest, but not for the stomach, as he prescribed a severe and exacting master to stimulate the tired and overworked stomach to renewed life, and so give the nerves plenty of pure food, as they were in need of same. I then, after getting a ravenous hunger, weakened myself still more and became worse. My stomach felt numb and paralyzed, as did also my other internal organs, but this was put down against me as an illusion. So a professor of nervous diseases was called in consultation, owing to my many desires to die (as life had no sunshine, flowers, or music for me); I was simply living a living death of torture which these professors would have were illusions. My parents were then informed that I must be sent to an asylum, where I was for ten long weeks. They also told me that my feelings were illusions, and proceeded to banish the same by giving the tired-out nerves a little rest and plenty of nourishment on a five-meal plan per day. If refused (owing to a loss of appetite), I was threatened to have nature helped by the aid of a stomach or nasal tube. I lost none of my illusions while there, as I could not feel any improvement in my feelings. I left the institution June 28,

1899, feeling no better; in fact, worse than when I arrived there. I was then taken from one doctor to another, the one wishing to operate, the other not; one advising me to go to the seashore, country, etc., but none to give my stomach the needed vacation.

"'It was then that my friend, Mr. Ritter, stepped in, as he saw the failures of professors and specialists, and begged my parents to let him have a chance to demonstrate what Dr. Dewey's method would do for melancholy illusions and tired-out stomachs and nerves. I then went to friends, and, in entire ignorance of my parents, began under directions of Mr. Ritter the most natural, sensible, and cheapest of all cures. I began my fast on Oct. 3, and broke the same on Nov. 16. During the first week of my fast I was in bed; during the second (excepting the eleventh day, when I took my first walk of seven-eighths of a mile) I was in bed, in rocker, reading, etc. On the twentieth day, after a drive of three hours, went to church, walking two and one-sixteenth miles. I then stayed indoors again on the twenty-first and twenty-second days, and then started taking daily walks (weather permitting). I went out walking twenty-three out of the forty-five days of my fast, and during that time walked one hundred and twelve miles. This was besides the carriage-drives, Exposition, and evening gatherings (walking to same included). I did not in the least feel tired or weak, but happier and brighter each day of the fast, as I could feel the effects of a new life throughout my whole body. My mind also became clearer and dizziness became a thing of the past. This was indeed joy supreme to me, and life became once more a joy instead of a burden. Sunshine, trees, flowers, etc., again made an impression, and my parents, sisters, and friends are rejoiced to see me in my happy normal state of health.

"'I have gone through a year of unspeakable torture brought on by overwork and human-wise professors; but at last, through the wonderful teachings Dr. Dewey has given to mankind, and through a friend, who was able to preach the "New Gospel of Health," am now well, strong, and happy. May God only help and bless the many sufferers throughout the world (especially in the asylums) with the rays of this Gospel. I have been saved, no doubt, from a gloomy future, and may such be the realization of many more unfortunate souls is the sincere wish through experience of

"'Yours very sincerely,

"'ESTELLA F. KUENZEL.'"

This case was summed up in the Philadelphia Public Ledger of Dec. 25, 1899, whose columns are guarded with unsurpassed care, as follows:

"One of those cases which a judicious editor ponders in no little perplexity is that of a young lady who was taken out of an insane hospital and subjected to a protracted fast, without medical supervision, and with results that appear to have been quite successful. On the one hand, there is the benefit that may be derived by having the attention of the profession called to the subject, with possibly good results; on the other hand, there is the danger of having a lot of ignorant or impulsive people risking their lives by starving themselves for this or that real or fancied disease, forgetting the adage that a little knowledge is a dangerous thing, especially in therapeutics.

"The mind of the young lady referred to became affected about a year ago, and after what was regarded by her parents as an unprofitable period of treatment for two and a half months in a hospital for the insane she has been apparently cured by fasting--some would call it starvation. The case has been attracting attention and discussion lately in a growing circle that has included a few physicians.

"The subject is a Miss K., aged twenty-two years. Henry Ritter, who has charge of the Photography Department of the Drexel Institute, and who is better acquainted with the matter than any one else, furnished a Ledger reporter with the particulars as they are here given, the name and address of the young lady, for obvious reasons, being omitted. Mr. Ritter was at first loath to have any publicity given the case, but felt upon reflection that the results were properly a subject matter for inquiry by physicians, at least, not to speak of others who may be interested.

"Miss K., by the advice of specialists who had treated her at home, was put under treatment for melancholy in an institution for the insane. Mr. Ritter, being an intimate friend of the family, visited her, and, he says, found her retrograding. She was receiving three meals a day, with two luncheons between them. Having built up his own digestive powers by following the tenets laid down by Dr. Dewey, a Crawford county physician, he had become a student and advocate of the latter's theory, briefly stated, that no food should be given to a patient except in response to a natural call or appetite for it. Believing that no improvement could result from the course Miss K. was receiving in the hospital, he prevailed upon her parents to permit him to have her placed in the home of a friend, and suggested the fasting process. This was the more readily done as the physicians in whose care she had been advised her parents to leave their daughter as much as possible among strangers.

"This young lady, according to Mr. Ritter, was absolutely without food for forty-five days, beginning October 3 and ending November 16. He says he did not fear, as others did, that she would starve, as the authority he depended on had never fed a sick patient during a practice covering twenty-two years, no matter how protracted the case might have been, and claimed to have had only the best results. 'This,' said Mr. Ritter, 'is on the theory that, since all bodily energy is the result of the brain, by abstaining from feeding in the absence of appetite there is all the energy of cure undiverted by needless waste in the stomach. Feeding the sick, this physician contends, is a tax on their vital power, adding indigestion to whatever other troubles exist: because the brain has the power in sickness to absorb nourishment from the body, as predigested food, so that it never loses weight, even in death from starvation.'

"The patient herself became interested, Mr. Ritter says, and evidenced great relief from abstinence from enforced periodic feeding. Gradually a numb feeling of which she had complained as affecting her internal organs, and which had been ascribed to her illusions, left her, and she appeared to gain daily in strength and brightness. Mr. Ritter's narrative proceeds:

"'On the eleventh day of her fast a walk was suggested, and she covered about seven-eighths of a mile; on the twentieth day she was taken for a carriage drive of three hours in the afternoon, and in the evening she walked to church and back, a distance of something more than two miles. From the twenty-third day she took walks daily, excepting on October 31 and November 3, when rain prevented. She visited friends and the theatre and the Exposition, went to church several times, to the hospital where she had been a patient--this on the thirty-fifth day of her fast--and to the Drexel Institute on the thirty-ninth and forty-second days. A table of dates shows that she walked from two or three to six and eight and as high as nine miles a day during the period of forty-five days that she abstained from food, with a general increase of strength and cheer and no sign of fatigue. Hunger sensations were marked on the forty-fourth day and night, and on the morning of the forty-fifth day Miss K. broke the fast by eating a poached egg and two slices of buttered whole wheat toasted bread.

"'During her fast she was seen by seven physicians and medical professors, President MacAlister and professors of the Drexel Institute, and many others.'

"The young lady's weight at the beginning of the fast, Mr. Ritter says, was one hundred and forty pounds, and just after the meal with which she broke the fast she weighed one hundred and twenty pounds. By December 15 she had regained nine pounds, meanwhile eating one meal daily and sometimes two, with an occasional light luncheon.

"Dr. Chase, medical director of the institution above referred to, was visited on Saturday by a Ledger reporter in regard to the case of Miss K. He had been informed of her long fast and of its results, and had seen Miss K. herself when she called at the asylum on the thirty-fifth day of the fast. He said that when she was first brought to the asylum she was suffering from melancholia, and was put under the treatment which all the leading alienists had found most beneficial for persons suffering from nervous disorders, viz., quiet, rest of mind and body, and full, nourishing diet, carefully selected to produce the best results. During the time she remained at the asylum she improved both in bodily and mental health.

"Referring to the treatment she had received under Mr. Ritter's supervision since leaving the asylum, Dr. Chase said he had first heard of the system through a work published two years ago by Dr. George S. Keith, of London, from which he first learned of Dr. Dewey, who also uses the fasting cure. In all the cases cited by Dr. Keith none had been afflicted with any mental disorder. He looked upon the cases, however, as showing some remarkable results, warranting a careful study. But it would not do to adopt such a system without a most thorough examination. As 'one swallow does not make a summer,' neither will one case nor half a dozen cases cured by such a method prove anything. No universal method can be adopted for treating disease. Hardly two cases are alike. Cures also may be brought about in different ways if the exact condition of the patient is understood.

"'Mr. Ritter says the patient lent herself very willingly to the treatment, which was a great deal to start out with in her case. But I am surprised that a young man with no medical knowledge would do a thing like that. The treatment might easily have resulted differently. If he had been a doctor, he would have had that fact to sustain him in case he got into trouble. The case might very well have resulted fatally, because the treatment was so contrary to what would naturally be pursued by physicians in nervous cases.

"'I do not ridicule the system. There have been cases which were cured by ways not recognized by the general practitioner after they had been given up. I am a firm believer that in selected cases the fasting method would be efficacious, but I do not believe in its general application.

"'Mr. Ritter is evidently an enthusiast, and apt to overstate the points in favor of the method, neglecting those which tell against it. It is too early yet to say what the outcome of Miss K.'s case will be. I think the matter ought to be looked into more fully. Mr. Ritter could not have been with the patient at all times. It is a remarkable thing that she should have kept up and had the strength reported, unless she had some food. He may have been deceived in that.'"

During several months since the fast there have been the best physical health and mental condition, the weight having increased several pounds above the former average.

Mr. Ritter conducted this case in a blaze of publicity. He showed it to no less than seven physicians, some of whom were college professors, and one of them at near the close of the fast suggested that if food were not soon taken a sudden collapse would be the result. There seemed to have been less danger of this calamity on the forty-fourth day than on any other.

The reliability of the fast was so clearly evident that the leading papers of the city accepted it as authentic news and of the most startling kind. The Times gave several columns of its first page to an illustrated article.[1]

The accompanying illustration shows Miss Kuenzel on the forty-first day of her fast. She walked seven miles on this day without any signs of fatigue.

The following table of miles walked were measured from exact diary notes with bicycle and cyclometer after the fast was broken. The table gives the total sum of each day, walks being taken both afternoon and evenings of same day.

Date. Miles.

October 3 " 4 " 5 " 6 " 7 " 8 " 9 " 10 " 11 " 12 " 13 7/8 " 14 " 15 " 16 " 17 " 18 " 19 " 20 " 21 " 22 2-1/16 " 23 " 24 " 25 3 " 26 6-5/8 " 27 5-7/8 " 28 4-1/2 " 29 4-1/8 " 30 5-5/8 " 31, rain November 1 6-3/4 " 2 8 " 3 rain " 4 9 " 5 6 " 6 3-3/4 " 7 1-1/2 " 8 7-1/4 " 9 7 " 10 4-1/4 " 11 2-5/8 " 12 7 " 13 2-1/4 " 14 3-1/4 " 15 5 " 16 5-3/4 -------- 112-1/16

The next fast, under the care of Mr. Ritter, still holds the record as being the most remarkable for its number of days and the miracle of results. The following account of it appeared in the North American, one of whose editors had personal knowledge of its history:

"Leonard Thress, of 2618 Frankford Avenue, has learned how to live without eating. By physical experience he has proved not only that food is not a daily necessity of the human system, but that abstinence therefrom for protracted periods is beneficial. Indeed, it saved his life. He has just finished a fifty days' fast. When he began it he was on the brink of the grave and his physicians had abandoned hope. When he ended it he was in better health than he had enjoyed for years, although in the meantime he had lost seventy-six pounds, falling away from two hundred and nine to one hundred and thirty-three pounds.

"Thress, who is about fifty-seven years old, was attending the Grand Army Encampment at Buffalo in the fall of 1898, when he caught a violent cold, which settled in his bronchial tubes. It proved so stubborn that his general health became affected, and a year later dropsy developed. His condition grew steadily worse, and at Christmas time, 1899, it was such that he could neither walk nor lie prostrate, but was compelled to sit constantly in an armchair. His doctors exhausted their skill in the effort to bring relief, and eventually, in the early part of last January, they told him that their medicines refused to act, and that his death was a question of only a few days.

"Up to this time Thress had been subsisting on the meagre diet permitted to a man in his condition, but his stomach rebelled even at that. He had heard of the Dewey fasting cure and its boasted efficacy against all human ills, and, though he had little faith, death was already looming before him, and he knew that he could lose nothing by the experiment.

"He began to fast on January 11 by taking in the morning a portion of Henzel's preparation of salts in a glass of water and the juice of two oranges, and in the evening a hot lemonade. For twenty-five days he also drank a teaspoonful of a tonic consisting chiefly of iron, but the rest of the diet he continued until two weeks ago, when he discontinued the salts and orange juice and confined himself to a hot lemonade at morning and evening. This was his only sustenance until last Thursday.

"According to Thress's own recital, the effects of this course of treatment were amazing. He says that the natural craving for food was gone after the first day. Three days later he had regained so much strength that he was able to go upstairs to bed and enjoyed a good night's sleep. From that time on, although he steadily lost in weight, his vitality grew greater, and on January 22 he left the house and took a half-mile walk.

"Before three weeks of his fast had elapsed his dropsy had disappeared, and thereafter he took almost daily walks, increasing the distance with his strength. Some days he covered as many as five miles, and never less than two, even while he was growing thinner and thinner, as the accompanying table shows.

"For the first time since the beginning of his fast he became hungry last Thursday, March 1, and he felt that he should like some pigs' feet jelly. It is one of the prescriptions of the fasting cure that when hunger finally comes the patient shall eat whatever he craves, so Thress consumed two slices of the jelly and one piece of gluten bread, with butter. He says he enjoyed it and felt well afterward.

"He ate no more that day, but at noon yesterday he became hungry again, and this time his appetite was for something more substantial. He disposed of a dish of mashed potatoes, some red cabbage, another portion of pigs' feet jelly, apple sauce, and a cream puff for dessert. He even smoked a cigar after the meal, enjoyed it, and felt still better. He says he will eat no regular meals, but only when he becomes hungry.

"While he looks haggard and worn from the loss of flesh, Thress declares that all his ailments have left him and that he never felt healthier and heartier in his life."

* * * * *

"The following table shows how Thress grew stronger and walked miles while he was constantly losing weight from a fifty-days' fast:

Weight. January 11 209 " 12 207 " 13 205 " 14 202 " 15 201 " 16 200 " 17 199 " 18 196 " 19 192 " 20 190 " 21 188 " 22 186 Walked 1/2 mile. " 23 180 " 2 miles. " 24 177 " 2 " " 25 172 " 3 " " 26 167 " 3 " " 27 165 " 3 " " 28 162 " 2-1/2 " " 29 160 " 3 " " 30 157 " 31 155 " 3 " February 1 154 " 2 153 " 3 152 " 3 " " 4 151 " 5 149 " 3 " " 6 147 " 3 " " 7 146 " 3 " " 8 145 " 9 145 " 4 " " 10 145 " 4 " " 11 145 " 12 145 " 4 " " 13 145 " 14 145 " 3 " " 15 144 " 2 " " 16 142 " 17 140 " 18 140 " 19 140 " 20 138 " 2 " " 21 137 " 4 " " 22 135 Walked 3 miles. " 23 135 " 3 " " 24 135 " 25 135 " 26 135 " 27 133 " 2 " " 28 133 March 1 133

A. H. Potts, Editor of the Chester County Times, a man who has the largest faith in eating only to restore the wastes of the body, thus gives vent to his emotions after seeing the case by invitation of Mr. Ritter:

"On January 10 there sat in his home, at 2618 Frankford Avenue, Philadelphia, Mr. Leonard Thress, with dropsy, hopelessly given up to a speedy death by the many physicians he had vainly sought and paid well for relief. His weight was two hundred and nine pounds. His limbs were at the bursting point, and the water was close up to the top of his chest. He could not lie down nor even lay his head back without choking, and to walk across the room completely exhausted him. At that critical moment a friend of his heard of Miss Kuenzel's miraculous cure, and told him of it. He at once sent for Mr. Ritter, who thought that a cure was in his reach, and on January 11 Thress commenced a fast that has been absolute up to yesterday, the only things passing his lips being water, a little lemonade, and rarely the juice of an orange. Learning through the Chester County Times that we were interested in Dr. Dewey's discovery, he invited us to come and see the cases now under his care, and on Friday of last week we gladly availed ourselves of the opportunity to see the living proof of what we believed but had never seen. We were very cordially received at Mr. Ritter's home, and instead of meeting a pompous, egotistic, big man, as we might expect, we met a young gentleman of small stature, like ourselves, modest, retiring, and claiming no credit for his own part in these remarkable cures; but insisting that he is only observing the progress of cases, following in the line of truths discovered only by Dr. Dewey, giving such advice as he is enabled to do from his thorough knowledge of chemistry, anatomy, and hygiene. He took us to the house of Mr. Thress, and the startling impressions we received can never be effaced. We seemed to be in the presence of one who had arisen from the dead, and could not realize the truth of what we saw and heard from him and his estimable wife, who shows the happiness she feels in receiving her husband back to life. Impossible as it seems, yet on the previous day, as well as many other days, that man had walked three miles after six hours given to his business as a baker, which he now attends to personally. All traces of dropsy have disappeared, and his weight is now less than one hundred and thirty-five pounds, having lost this nearly seventy-five pounds of water through the natural channels at the rate of five or six pounds per day at times. His eyesight has grown younger and his hand is firm. He sleeps soundly several hours out of each twenty-four, and is almost a cured man, although the curative action is still going forward throughout his system, and his many friends are now awaiting the arrival of his normal healthy appetite, which in these cases does not arrive until the cure is entire, and then it comes in such a way as not to be mistaken. On Monday of this week we again visited him, taking a friend who has long suffered similarly to what he did, that she might see results for herself. We found him looking even better than on Friday, and it is very interesting to hear him tell his experience, which he will be glad to impart to those who are seeking after the truth, and interested in the cure of disease of themselves or their friends by this natural and without price (but priceless) means. We also visited two other of the five cases over which Mr. Ritter is at present keeping watch, and every one bore evidences of the great truth. No one should undertake the fast on their own responsibility, as certain conditions may arise requiring the eye of one who has made the matter a study, and no one should pass an opinion on the matter until they read Dr. Dewey's New Gospel of Health, wherein the reasons are made so plain that all can understand."

Mr. Thress has regained his normal weight and has been in the best of health in the several months since the fast.[2]

The following case was deemed a miracle by all friends: Mrs. H. B., a woman of seventy-six, became exceedingly breathless, due, it was supposed, to defective heart action that had been chronic for many years. The final result was general dropsy. The eyelids had become so heavy that reading could be indulged only a short time because of their weight; the throat was also charged with water so as to make swallowing difficult. Beneath the eyes and jaws were pockets of water--in short, the skin of the entire body was distended, a condition that had deceived the friends as revealing only an increase of her natural stoutness. The real condition became known through a call to treat a bad cold.

What had authorized medical art to promise in such a case? Absolutely nothing, as she had become too old and weak to be subjected to the ordinary means for such a general condition. As for a fast for one so old, that was the last thing that would have been thought of: her age and debility would only have seemed to invite more daily food than she had been taking.

She was put on a fast, or rather the fast was continued, the cold having abolished her appetite. It went on until the fifteenth day, with increasing general strength and diminishing weight. The last days before hunger came she was able to go up a long flight of stairs without the aid of the railing and without marked loss of breath, the heart-murmur had nearly disappeared, and water by the gallon seemed to have been absorbed.

On the fifteenth day there was a desire for food, that was taken with relish through the enlarged throat without difficulty; the water pockets had become emptied, and the lids so thin and light as to reveal no fatigue in reading. Thence on one meal a day became the rule; and since there have been five years without any recurrence of the conditions--five years of remarkable general health and girl-time relish for her daily food.

How often has the cutting down of the daily food by the old and weak been condemned as too severe an ordeal to be safe! For this woman there have been these acquired years of nearly perfect health, and the end will be in the natural, easier death of old age.

The following is inserted as additional evidence of Nature's power over disease, and that brain-workers may go on with their labors with increasing power while waiting for natural hunger in cases in which hunger is possible:

Rev. C. H. Dalrymple, of Hampden, Mass., has just completed a fast, of which he says, February 5, 1900: "My fast continued thirty-nine and one-half days. My appetite came on me about 9 o'clock at night, and I thought I would wait until the next day; but two boiled eggs and some dry toast would not retire before my presence. I have never had such an assault upon my will power as that imagined egg and toast made on me. I was finally compelled to surrender. My tongue had been clearing up that day, and the next day I was hungry at noon. I have not missed a first-class appetite at noon since. My tongue has kept clear and my taste has remained sweet. I have had no chills nor fevers this winter, nor cold in any form. I have made no allowance for my sickness and have never worked harder. My flesh came back rapidly, and now I think I must weigh about fifteen pounds more than last summer. I gained strength beyond all question about three weeks before my appetite returned. I would work all day long finally. It was good to get well."

Mr. Ritter conducted over twenty cases, some being able to carry on their usual avocations. I give the most important ones: Mr. A. H., forty-five days; Miss B. H., forty-two days; Mrs. L., thirty-eight days; Mr. L. W., thirty-six days; Miss L. J., thirty-five days; Mrs. M., thirty-one days; Miss E. S., twenty-six days; Mr. G. R., twenty-five days; Mr. P. R., twenty-four days; and Miss E. Westing, forty-two days, who, on the fortieth day, was able to sing with unusual clearness and power, and ended her fast without losing a day from her duties as a teacher of music.[3]

Wonderful are these fasts? Not in the physiological sense. These fasts went on with only increasing comfort by day and more refreshing sleep at night. It is quite another thing to endure the fasts of acute sickness, for such they all are. That life is maintained for days and weeks, even months, under pain, discomfort--under all the torturing conditions of such diseases as pneumonia, typhoid fever, or inflammatory rheumatism, is far more a matter to wonder over.

I may well wonder that Nature is powerful enough to cure the sick at all even under the wisest aid; but with me the abiding wonder is that physicians do not see that acute sickness is a loss of all the natural conditions of digestion, with the wasting bodies the clearest evidence that food is neither digested nor assimilated. I wonder with only increasing impatience that the stomach is not understood as a machine that Nature wills shall not be run to tax her resources when life is in the throes of disease.

MISS ELIZABETH W. A. WESTING,

FORTIETH DAY OF FAST.]

FOOTNOTES:

[1] The fasts conducted by Mr. Ritter constitute performances of the most impressive kind as demonstrative evidence of the practical physiology I have been teaching for many years. For the copyrighted photographs he has kindly furnished I am very thankful, and to all who have been willing to enhance the value and interest of this volume by such eyesight illustrations.

[2] The accompanying illustration shows Mr. Thress on the fiftieth day of his fast; weight loss, seventy-six pounds. Does the picture reveal any skeleton condition?

[3] The accompanying illustration is a reproduced copyrighted picture of Miss E. Westing. This picture was taken on the return home from her duties at church on the fortieth day during the cold of winter; the weight at the start being one hundred and ten pounds, at the close on the forty-second day ninety-three pounds--loss, seventeen pounds.

XIII.

I had not been long engaged in observing the evolution of cure through Nature when I began to suspect strongly, as before intimated, that fasting is the true "medicine for the mind diseased." Not less evident than the cure of various ailings would be the emergence of the soul into higher life, and in some instances from the depth of despair. As the scope of my vision constantly enlarged through multiplying experiences, I began to see great hopes of the cure of the gravest of all diseases--insanity--through a rigid application of this method in Nature. I gave the matter so much thought and study that I wrote a monograph on the subject with the idea of publishing it, but gave it up to the idea of telling my impressions in "The No-breakfast Plan."

There are the same structural changes in the evolution of insanity as in that of catarrh. There is a morbid structural basis in minds diseased, the abnormal mentality or morality being merely symptoms of a physical disease. Of all human legacies, structural weakness of the mental or moral sense is the most unfortunate.

I shall say no more about the forms of mental disease than that there is distinctively both intellectual and moral insanity as a direct result of disease of the intellectual and moral centres. This will be more clearly seen when I recall the fact that moral insanity in its worse form--the suicidal--often exists with such intellectual clearness that there is the greatest ingenuity displayed in carrying out self-destruction. These mind and soul centres are often gravely diseased without impairment of muscle energy: the furious strength of the insane is an abiding fear with all.

It is clear that weakness of structure so soft as brain, a substance which is on the dividing-line between liquids and solids, must be of the gravest form from the first: grave because so fragile, grave because the sick centres cannot rest as the broken arm, the sick body: these centres, regardless how sick, must continue to serve, even in abnormal ways.

The possibility of insanity must always be a matter of the degree of the primary structural weakness and the energy and persistence of the operative forces; on these must depend the mere gentle, persistent illusion, or that fury of mania which transforms man, the "image of the Creator," into a wild beast. That insanity, no matter what its form or degree, is an evolution from an ancestral structural legacy, not essentially different from the structural conditions evolved from those of any other chronic disease, I cannot have the slightest doubt, any more than I can have for the structural means for the cure.

There is nothing that so illustrates the civilization, the benevolence of the age and of the nations as these palaces we call hospitals for the insane. Whatever there is that can add comfort to the body, or charm to the tastes, or new life to the soul has its culmination in these palaces of wood and stone, with one great exception: the structural condition of the diseased centres indicating rest, even as the ulcer, wound, or fracture, has no part in the methods of cure.

The feeding is all done not at the time of hunger, but at the time of day. All patients are expected to eat no less than three meals a day, regardless of any desire for food and whether the patient spends all his time in bed in mindless apathy, whether pacing his room with meaningless tread, whether active in light service in the building or in heavy labor without. When there is refusal to eat it seems to be taken for granted that suicide by starvation is the design, and the pumping of food into the stomach through the nose is the common resort. There seems to be no thought that there may be no hunger in such cases, and no apprehension of any danger from not eating; that in this they follow the instincts of brutes. Would the desire for food not come and with a saner condition of mind if they were permitted their own ways of eating?

A physically strong woman, whom I knew well, was sent to a hospital for the insane in a generally bad state of mind, with destructive propensities marked. With no desire for food, and certainly with no mind to realize the need to eat without hunger, she naturally refused to eat. But for a time her meals were forced down her throat, a proceeding that taxed the strength of several strong arms.

Why were the meals not omitted long enough to cause such a reduction of strength as to make feeding less expensive in the outlay of others' muscle? The persistent refusal to eat resulted in a cessation of all efforts to enforce food; left to the gentler hands of Nature for a time, the mental hurricane subsided in great degree on the return of hunger, and long before there was an appreciable loss of weight or strength. In a few months this woman was able to return to her home, and with restored mind to tell me of the violent feedings she had endured.

Now let us look again to the structural conditions involved in diseases of the mind. There are those soft, pulpy centres from which emanate the highest powers of life: power to think, to admire, to rejoice, or to suffer; and we know how digestive power varies along the scale between ecstacy and despair. In mental disease there is the same abnormal structural change as in other local diseases; but for these sick mind-centres there is no rest. There must be still thinking and feeling, no matter how chaotic, to tax them, and there is no cheer to electrify the stomach into easy display of power. We may well marvel that powers so wonderful as the power to think, love, admire, see, hear, and feel are located in structures so fragile as the brain; and we may well marvel at the provision of the turret of flinty hardness to protect it from violence.

Now we are to consider these centres of energy as abnormally weak in all their structures at birth in those who become insane: these are the luckless legacies from the fathers and the mothers, and for how far back in the ancestral line we do not know. We are to consider that there is the same abnormal condition of the cerebral bloodvessels and of the softer intervascular structures as in other local diseases; and when you recall the fact that everything that worries, that adds discomfort to either mind or muscles, is a force that tends to develop weakness and disease, you will see how it applies in the evolution of insanity.

Shall these fragile centres be permitted to rest when overwork has made them sick, or is there any other rational means for their recovery? Shall they not be permitted to rest when abundantly able to keep physically nourished in a way that does not cause even the slightest shade of discomfort?

Again, let it be borne in mind that recovery from acute disease is attended with a revival of strength in every power that makes life worth living, and that every person not acutely sick who has fasted under my care or who has cut down the waste of brain power by less daily food has found the same revival of power. To this there have been no exceptions.

What do we fear in sickness? Is it disease or the wasting pounds? Since they will disappear when Nature would have the food-gate closed, since they reappear when there is the highest possible reach of mere relish, and when all the other senses have become more acute, and also when existence has become almost ecstatic, why ever oppress the weak or sick centres when Nature wills a rest?

The literature on the disease of the mind has become so massive in mere bulk, in its physiological refinements, that it would require time with a long reach into eternity to go through it; but it has not come to my knowledge that it contains any reference to the brain as a self-nourishing, self-charging dynamo; that therefore the stomach is only a machine whose use can well be omitted for long periods when these centres of moral and intellectual energy have become worried into disease, with rest the only means, the only need for all the recovery possible.

"Oh, you giants of the medical profession!" You who have been elected to preside over these great homes of the mentally wrecked because of your eminence in character, ability, experience, and professional attainments, do you deny the soundness of the physiology involved in this method of reaching health through Nature? Then let me array against you Alexander Haig, M. A., M. D. Oxon., F. R. C. P., Physician to the Metropolitan Hospital, and the Royal Hospital, and for Children and Women; late Casualty Physician to St. Bartholomew's Hospital. I quote from his exhaustive work, Uric Acid in the Causation of Disease:

"And now I come to the causes which led me to take too much albumen and to suffer severely; in Fads of an Old Physician, Dr. Keith refers to another work on diet, by Dr. Dewey, of Meadville, Pa., The True Science of Living, and the chief point in this book is that temporary, complete starvation till there is once more a healthy appetite is the best cure for a host of dyspepsia, debilities, depression, mental and bodily, and numerous other troubles, and that for similar less severe disturbances of nutrition the great remedy is to leave out the breakfast, so as to give the stomach a long rest of sixteen hours or more, with the object of allowing it to recuperate and accumulate secretions after the last meal of the previous day.

"It seems from internal evidence in Dr. Dewey's book, a copy of which I owe to Dr. Keith, that his plans have been completely successful in a large number of cases, and it seems to me that his logic is unanswerable, and that in his main contentions he is perfectly right.

"Having arrived at this conclusion, I proceeded forthwith to put the matter to the test of experience by placing myself on two meals a day--that is, I left out my breakfast--and the result was I ate such a good lunch at 1 P. M. that it was impossible to take anything more till dinner-time, 7.30 or 8 P. M.; so that I reduced myself at once from four meals a day to two. The result was exactly what Dr. Dewey describes. I felt extremely bright and well in the morning, and capable of very good work, both mental and bodily. At 1 P. M. I had keen hunger, even for dry bread; such hunger as I had not experienced for years. After lunch (breakfast) I felt a little bit dull and occasionally sleepy, and the mental work for the first hour or two after it was not as good as usual. About 5 P. M. I was very thirsty and had to have a drink of water, but there was not the least desire for food until several hours later; though by 7.30 or 8 P. M. I was able to manage another fairly good meal; and thus my meals automatically, so to speak, reduced themselves to two."

I also quote from his work on Diet and Food, page 10:

"It is also possible, by introducing more food than can possibly be digested, to overpower digestion so that nothing is digested and absorbed, and starvation results, a fact that has been brought to the front in the most interesting manner in the writings of Dr. Dewey."

And who is Dr. Keith? You know that he is one of the youngest physicians in all Scotland, even if he does possess eighty years that are no burden to him. I quote him from his Fads of an Old Physician:

"Dr. Dewey's grand means of cure now is abstinence for the time from all food, and this he carries out to a degree which must astonish most physicians of the present day, as well as their patients. During times of sickness, when there is no desire for food, he gives none till the desire comes, and then only if the state of the tongue and general condition show that the power of digestion has returned. This may be in a few days, or in severe cases, as of rheumatic fever, it may not be for forty days or even longer. He points out very forcibly that we have all a store of material laid up in the body which supplies what is required for keeping necessary functions of the system going, while no food can be usefully taken in the stomach. I had mentioned this provision in my Plea, and had stated that so long as it lasts it is sufficient to preserve life. I also suggested that it might be found that the waste of the body was less when this internal supply was alone trusted to, than when it was supplemented by food from without which the organs of nutrition were not in a condition to utilize. This, to my mind, Dr. Dewey has proved to be the fact, and no one can read his case without being convinced that it is so. He gives a most interesting table from Dr. Yeo, showing what textures of the body waste most rapidly in disease. Fat is at one end of the scale, and at the other the brain, which does not waste till all the other textures and organs are depleted to the utmost.

"In cases of slighter disease where the patient is able to be about or to carry on his business, but with discomfort, the same abstinence from all food is recommended. It is usually found that work can be done more easily, and that strength actually increases, although the starving may have to be kept up for several days. But the great coup in Dr. Dewey's practice is, that to improve or to preserve health he advises all to give up breakfast, and to fast till the mid-day meal. In this he has had a very large number of followers, very much to their advantage. It may be that the omission of breakfast is more needed and has greater effect in America than it would have on this side of the Atlantic. In America the meal is generally a very full one, made up in a large measure of a variety of hot cakes, also flesh food and tea or coffee. The other two meals of the day are full, 'square' meals likewise. I have seen much overfeeding in this country, but never to such a degree, and so generally, as I have seen in America and on American steamers. In one of the latter the cooking was the worst I ever met with, but the hard meat was swallowed all the same, and the consequences must have been grievous."

Are you still without any questioning of your authorized, established methods of treating the mentally sick? Then let me quote against you another man across the ocean, whose ability, learning, and professional attainments are of the highest order. I quote from Air, Food, and Exercise, by A. Rabagliati, M. A., M. D., F. R. C. S., Edin., a man with whom patient, exhaustive investigation is only a recreation:

"It has been shown by physiologists that certain tissues are absorbed and used before others. Dr. Dewey, of Pennsylvania, with whose views I am glad to find myself in general accord, and who seems to have made the same attempt as the writer to view the facts of medical practice from an independent--and may I say, original?--standpoint, quotes a table of great significance from Dr. Yeo. Besides quoting it in the text of his book, The True Science of Living, Dr. Dewey places it in capital letters in the frontispiece of his book. He calls it Nature's Bill of Fare for the Sick; and he shows that in illness, when we are using up the materials accumulated in our bodies, we may use as much as 99 per cent. of our fat (practically all of it), that of muscle we may use as much as 30 per cent., that the spleen may waste to the extent of 63 per cent., the liver as much as 56 per cent., and the blood itself be absorbed to the extent of 17 per cent. of its total amount. But even when wasting to this extent has occurred the curious and significant fact is emphasized that the brain and nerve-centres may not have wasted at all. The controlling nervous system thus does not lose its powers till the very last. Generally, however, the wasting process does not require to be carried to the very last, the chronic inflammatory deposit (and in rare cases even a cancerous infiltration) being absorbed and got rid of before this point is reached.

"As most, if not all, of the chronic diseases depend upon the deposition of waste, unassimilated materials in various situations; or, in other words, depend upon a blocking of the local circulation in this way, a little wholesome starvation is generally of vast benefit by inducing the economy to use up some of its waste stuff. Nature herself points the way to us in this matter, because when things have gone as far as she can bear, and when, were things to go on in the same way, death must ensue, she generally throws the patient into bed with a digestive system entirely disorganized, taking away all appetite for food and all power of assimilation for the time being. We may, in such circumstances, do much harm by efforts too persistently made to feed our patients; but generally they refuse all sustenance for some time. After a while (Dr. Dewey does not seem to be afraid if his patients refuse all food even for as long on some occasions as thirty days continuously, or even longer) they right themselves, the tongue cleans, appetite returns, the power of assimilation is reestablished, and recovery takes place. It strikes me as somewhat curious (and yet, if we both look at the facts of life candidly and impartially, perhaps it is not curious) that observers so wide apart, and in circumstances so very different as the conditions of human life must be in Yorkshire from what they are in Pennsylvania, should come to conclusions so practically similar as Dr. Dewey and the writer have reached."

Gentlemen, masters in the medical profession, to what good end are you pumping food into human stomach, where there is no hunger and no mind left to know the need? Is it to maintain that strength which costs you so much muscle at every feeding. Or is it that it would be a danger to lose a few pounds of body while Nature gets ready to ask for food in the gentlest and most persuasive way? Whatever there is in appeal to the best in any human life to uplift it from the deepest depths, you have at the readiest command. You seem amply equipped to reach everything but those sick, afflicted, oppressed brain-centres. You treat everything but these, but to these you are worse than the Egyptian task-masters in that you force needless labor where rest alone is the need. It is not bricks without straw, but labor with exhausted power; and for all your efforts you simply maintain weight at a tremendous cost to the energy of cure. In no class of patients is rest for the brain more indicated than in yours; in none are the means so at command and the results for good so promising. With your patients the importance of time for business or social use is no more a concern; the abnormal is all due to disease.

Let us consider those rooms of bedlam you call the "excitable wards." They who enter leave all hope (of the friends) behind. Is there special need in these regions of despair and mental chaos that the mere pounds and strength shall be kept up? What will be lost by protracted fasts? Nothing in the kitchen. As for the brain and those sick centres, they will feed themselves until the last heart-beat sends the last available nourishment to the remotest cell. Will the functions of the brain grow more abnormal by a suspension of digestive drafts upon it? Does rest to anything that is tired tend to the abnormal?

Again I ask, What will be lost by protracted fasts in such cases? Nothing but weight, of which the fat will be by far the larger part. Would there be worry about starvation? With most of the cases there is not mind enough to worry over anything from the standpoint of reason. The very fact of the absence of the sense of the importance of daily food would render fasts in the highest degree practical and successful.

The fasts could be instituted with the certainty of a calmer condition of mind as soon as the digestive tract would cease to call upon the brain for power, and with the probability that a surprising degree of improvement would be manifest in all, and long before the available body-food for the brain would be exhausted.

Gentlemen, you have treated acute sickness in all its forms, and you have had many cases in which, because of irritable stomachs, neither food nor medicine could be given. Day after day you have seen the wasting of the bodies, and you have also seen mental aberration or stupor lessen day by day as the disease lessened its grasp upon the brain-centres, and finally when the point of natural hunger was reached, you never found the lost pounds a matter of physical discomfort or mental abnormality or weakness; rather you have always found at this point a mental condition in every way the most highly satisfactory. I never saw brighter eyes, a happier expression on every line, than revealed by a woman after a fast of forty-four days, in which acute disease had reduced the weight forty pounds.

All overweight not due to dropsy or other disease is due to eating more food than the waste demands. As an abnormal condition overweight has received a great deal of attention in the way of misguided effort to both prevention and cure. These efforts are such conspicuous failures that even the patent medicine man has not found his "anti-fat nostrums" the happy means to fortune. There have been all kinds of limits built around bills of fare, but sooner or later Nature revolts and they are given up.

The reason that certain people take on weight easily and become "stout," is because of constitutional tendency, good digestion, and excess of food. As a general fact, the overweights are "large feeders," and they not only look well but feel well, for they have much less stomach trouble than the average mortal, and in cheerful endowment of soul they rank the highest among all the people.

In spite of my philosophy, I, who am one of the leanest of the kind, look upon the stoutness of those in the early prime of life with something of both envy and admiration; they seem so ideally conditioned to enjoy the best of all things on earth. But it is quite a serious matter when the muscles and brain have to deal with pounds in excess by the score, even as if the victim were doomed to wear clothes padded with so many pounds of shot.

Why some people take on fat easily even with the smallest of meals, why some of the largest eaters are of the leanest, are matters to talk about but not to know about. For my purpose it is sufficient that I assert that overweight can be prevented by an habitual limitation of the daily food to the daily need; that it can be cut down to any desired degree by stopping the supply, a method that is not attended with any violence to the constitution, nor even to comfort or power. This plan has the great advantage of adding to the curative energy of disease as well; and more than this, there is a change attending the loss that seems at first phenomenal, as involving a physiological contradiction--there is an actual increase in muscle-weight as the bloat and fat weight go down.

How is this, you ask? Here is the explanation: As the fat weight increases by surplus food, so decrease the disposition and ability for general exercise. As it declines, so do muscle and all the other energies increase, and the use of muscle within physiological limit tends to restore the normal weight and strength.

There are no overweights who would not receive the greatest benefit by a fast that would diminish the pounds to that of the ripest maturity of life, a fast that would be determined by the time required to reach the desired number of pounds. As a means this method is available to all, and practical where due physiological light will enable it to be carried out with no starving concern to disable vital power.

As a general fact, the No-breakfast Plan has been attended by a highly satisfactory reduction of surplus pounds; where there has been a failure it has been due to such an increase of digestive power as really to add to both an increase of the average amount of daily food and of power to digest it. For instance, one of my fellow citizens, weighing not less than three hundred and thirty pounds some years ago, gave up his morning meals. This was attended with entire relief from frequent bilious spells; but the average of daily food was increased and the business of a barber did not add anything to muscle development. Finally from mere excess of weight he became a prisoner to his house and yard, unable to walk a square without the greatest difficulty; and yet there were two enormous meals put into a stomach daily that did not complain, and the weight increased until the three hundred and seventy-five pound notch was nearly reached. He heard about the Rathbun fast, and I was able to persuade him to come down to one light meal daily, and day after day bonds were loosened. After a year there have been nearly seventy-five pounds lost, and there is ability to labor and to walk several miles daily.

Very many thin persons have gained as high as forty pounds by reason of the larger degree of muscle exercise. Since last writing, this word has come from Miss K., who one year ago was at the asylum eating several meals a day in bed with suicidal intent. She left that bed with a weight of one hundred and forty pounds, and, as I have mentioned before, lost twenty pounds of it by her fast. My last news is from a letter written the day after a twenty-five-mile ride among the mountains with a soul as free and joyous as there are freedom and joy with the birds whose songs greeted her rapt ears from every treetop. She writes of a gain of twenty-four pounds since the fast, and states that the glasses she has worn for thirteen years are wanted no longer!

I feel that I need not multiply words as to the ability and utility of bringing all overweight down to the physiological normal and of keeping it there. I could fill hundreds of pages with the joyous testimonies of those who have been relieved of many surplus pounds, with numerous accompanying ailings; they all tell the same story, and I will only add this, that there is no physiological excuse for any mortal to carry around weight that disables.

Not very many months ago ex-Governor Flower, of New York, a statesman of national fame, a man of largest public spirit, a most valuable citizen, and Colonel Robert Ingersoll, an orator of world-wide fame and of great nobility of soul, dropped as beeves beneath the stroke of an ax because of a fracture of brittle bloodvessels. In both of these cases not many less pounds than a hundred had needlessly accumulated.

Could I have had the Colonel's ear when I last saw him as a listener to almost matchless oratory, whose rotundity of belt was to be measured by the yard, I would have addressed him as follows: "My dear Colonel, when I last saw you you were just filled out enough to be the joy of your tailor, and as a picture of health in form and looks you were ideal. You were then eating the meals of a woodchopper; and merely because food tastes good and does not seem to hurt you, you have been doing the same during the nearly score and a half of years since I have seen you. You have been eating more food every day in proportion to general muscle exercise than the hardest toiler does in a week, and your vast bulk evidences against you."

After explaining to him the structural possibilities of apoplexy as a legacy, as I have to you in the cases of insanity, I would continue: "Now by virtue of a possible ancestral weakness of your brain arteries this may happen: the arterial walls, because of habitual food in excess, may undergo a fatty, limy degeneration that will make a rupture possible, with death or paralysis of one-half or more of the body as the direct result; or the small arteries may have their walls so thickened as not to permit enough blood to circulate in order duly to nourish parts of the brain they supply; hence softening of the structure and more or less imbecility.

"The history of all overweights is that of a decline of muscle energy, and very generally of the amount of muscle activity as the pounds and years increase; but no cut in the amount of daily food so long as it can be taken with relish and disposed of without any special protesting from the stomach. This is the history of by far the largest majority of those sudden deaths due to cerebral hemorrhage, and also the history of most of the cases of imbecility with the overweights.

"Now, Colonel, you should make a radical parting with those surplus pounds by a fast that may extend into months, or take one of the lightest of meals once a day. Follow this out rigidly until you have lost a hundred pounds, and then by as much will you be not only free from disease, but free also from the danger of disease."

My experience with cases of epilepsy, or "fits," is confined to a half dozen cases, in which permanent relief seems to be assured. There is an acquired structural abnormality behind the spasms, acquired from surplus food, with a cure to be reached ultimately in most cases along these physiological lines.

XIV.

I shall not take time in telling the evils of alcoholics. It would not be more enlightening were I to spend hours in telling of wrecked lives, of wrecked homes, of prisons filled with their victims, of the immense loss to states and nations from the loss to sufferers and the loss they inflict. Alcoholism has no sense for frowning, ominous statistics, for it is a disease to be rationally treated, a disease to be rationally avoided.

In the light of later science the word "stimulants" has become a misnomer as applied to alcoholics; the term, no doubt, came into use from the fact that under their use there is more endurance to both physical and mental ills, an endurance or indifference ascribed to stimulation.

If power is stimulated by their use, then there should be a rise in temperature whereby severe cold is better endured; but this is not the fact any more than that temperature is lowered whereby extreme heat is endured; in either case the endurance is due to benumbed brain-centres. The alcoholic simply lessens the power to suffer mentally or physically; hence in degree it is an an æsthetic, and as such it also affects the moral sense and lessens the power of reason and judgment. They are habitually taken for no other reason than for the temporary relief they give to some ill of life.

It seems the very depths of total depravity when there is no bread for the hungry family, that the price of a loaf will rather be spent for a drink; but it is not so much moral depravity as depravity of brain-substance. The lethal drink is taken because without it there is more acute suffering than from the want of a loaf of bread by the entire family. In my practice an ordinarily sober father would always get drunk and stay drunk while any member of his family was sick, and for the sole reason that he could not endure the worry of apprehension. This was not so much depravity as an acute sense of the suffering and danger involved, a painful rousing of the best instincts of the soul, those instincts that raise man above the brute and make him the noblest work of the divine hand. That is not a bad man at heart who has such a sense of affection for his wife or child when they seem dangerously sick that he must have artificial aid to endurance; and if you shall detect the alcoholic odor in his breath at the funeral you may know that there is heart agony under repression.

The fact that alcoholics are an æsthetics, and not stimulants, has become known to a few of the scientists in the medical profession; but it can scarcely be said to have become known to the profession generally. That the habitual drinker partakes for any other reason than to drown his woes that will not stay drowned, and that the drowning is not stimulation, do not need argument.

The alcoholic in proportion to its strength is mental chaos and paralysis to power, and it has not the virtue to contain an atom that can be converted into a living atom. In not the least sense is it a tissue-builder, and its use by the medical profession is without the shadow of a reason, and is all the more reprehensible in cases of shock.

Let us see: shock in degree is brain paralysis; alcoholics in degree are brain paralyzers; shock is simply a state of exhaustion with rest the supreme need. All the rousement that is necessary and that can avail will be called into action by the need of oxygen. There are cases of disease in which breathing goes on hour after hour, when the soul seems to have departed and with it every life sense. The patient has become dead beyond reviving, and yet breathes hour after hour. Now can one for one moment think that an alcoholic can add to the power of the respiratory centres of the brain to respond to the calls for oxygen and so prolong life? Shock in its gravest degree is to be considered the extreme of the tired-out condition, with rest the only restorative means; and rest may be permitted with the certainty that for mere breathing purposes alcoholics are dangerous in proportion to the gravity of the shock.

In health the alcoholic only adds discomfort, because there are no complaints to soothe; hence it is the duty of every mother so to train her sons in health-habits that those first drinks will be discouraging because they bring no cheer of contrast, but rather sensations that are not suggestive of a better physical condition.

Alcoholics have a corroding effect upon the mucous membrane of the stomach, a congestive effect by which the glands are subjected to starving pressure; hence their use always disables the mere mechanics and the chemistry involved in digestion, and so prolongs disease, and this applies to all medicines that corrode. This corroding power of the alcoholics upon the walls of the stomach and its paralyzing effect upon the brain-centres, with the additional fact that there is nothing in it that adds force to any life power or that can be converted into living atoms, should make its use in the stomach of the sick a crime scarcely to be excused by ignorance.

The evolution of the drunkard is a process of culture, and involves something of a constitutional tendency as in other diseases. I conceive that there is an alcoholic temperament, or a temperament in which the inability to bear with patience the various mental and physical woes of life is marked even from childhood. Indigestion and every cause that lowers vital power only add to the importance of such a nervous system.

The first step in the evolution of the drunkard is the first untimely meal drawn from the breast of the mother. By irregular nursings and the nursings merely to stop crying the nervous system is continually overtaxed. There are the untimely meals to prevent gluttony; there are the between-meal lunches to incite nervousness, irritability, a feeling of unrest that nothing seems to satisfy.

This goes on year after year until the time comes when that first drink has power to soothe many discordant voices, and the die is cast. Other drinks follow, with each to lessen the power of the dynamo and to disable the machine. At first, drink is indulged not without a sense of wrongdoing, but with that feeling of power in reserve to keep within the limits of safety.

The gradual corrosion of the stomach adding to the labors of the brain in the matter of food mass decomposition as well as digestion marks the decline of power to abstain and the degradation of every sense that makes life worth living. Now add to the corrosion of the membrane and the paralysis of the brain-centres from alcoholics the other inciting causes in the culture of disease, and you have the evolution of the drunkard.

How is he to be cured? Only through a fast that shall let that diseased stomach become new from regeneration, that will let the brain accumulate rest in reserve. For a time you will need to have him under bonds, for his will power is abolished. Put him where there will be deaf ears to the cries of morbid nature, for there is to be a conflict at first; but long before hunger will come the storm will subside; and finally, when food will be really desired, there will be a new stomach and a new brain to which an alcoholic will be no temptation.

This is no figure of speech, because there is such a continual change of life and death going on in the soft tissues of the body that in a month or more of fasting it may be assumed that much of the tissues which is left has undergone reconstruction, and both brain and stomach act as if they are new when the time comes to restore the lost pounds.

The ways of the kitchen and dining-room are the ways of disease and death, ways whose ends are prisons, asylums, scaffolds, to a far larger extent than is dreamed of by the fathers and mothers of the land. A new crusade against intemperance, the intemperance of the dining-room, is the only one that will ever settle this so-called liquor question. The rum-seller will only pull down his sign through the starvation of his business.

With brains and stomachs kept in the highest order, the alcoholic has only the least power of the beguiling kind; it is rather a dose whose effects do not invite repetition. But for all who have the drink disease seemingly beyond hope a fast of a month, or two months if necessary, will cure any stomach or brain, no matter how pickled they are with alcoholic soaking, and with only the least disturbance in the habit breaking; even within a week the hardest of the fighting should be over when the fast is made absolute.

XV.

I have now to consider briefly a most distressing disease, one that perhaps was never cured by the power of doses, and that most happily illustrates the structural changes in the cure of disease.

Asthmatic distress is caused by congestion of the terminals of the bronchial tubes, by which entrance of air into the cells is made difficult, even in some cases to the point of suffocation. This condition as a disease may be called bronchial catarrh, as in most cases there is such a condition of the larger tubes as to cause the habitual raising of a discharge. As to the disease itself, you have only to recall what has been said about nasal catarrh in order to understand its origin and development. It would be as trivial a disease were it not for the fact that those smaller and ultimate tubes, because of flabby walls and weak vessels, become congested, with resulting narrowing of the air-ways of life.

For this most distressing disease local treatments are as futile and void of intelligence as the physiology and anatomy involved in cause and cure of other local diseases. Is it not a great thing that those too narrow ways of life may be reached through a fast which shall so charge the brain with power that the flabby walls will be condensed; that most cases of asthma may be cured, with marked relief for every case? This is as certain as a result, as that rest restores strength. With the toning of the brain through rest, a catarrh of the bronchial tubes is certainly curable in most cases. With a large opportunity to know I am able to say this with intense conviction.

Only a few months ago, just before the break of day, a freight train took a side track; in a few moments, with nearly a mile-a-minute speed, a limited passenger train took the same track, and in the time of a second five men were hurled into eternity. Why? How? The conductor and his brakeman were in such heavy sleep when the switch was opened that they were not awakened to close it.

Why? How? There was the torpor of indigestion holding the tired brains of those two men in its fatal grasp; their stomachs were full of food when they were already tired out by their long trip that was nearly at its close, and for them those untimely meals were the last.

Of all men who ought to work with empty stomachs for the sake of the best possible reach of the memory it is the railroad engineer and conductor; so also every man who is in any way responsible for the safety of the trains. If we had the history of all the derailments, collisions, of cars with human freight converted into funeral pyres, a frightful percentage of them could be traced to where "some one had blundered" because of the torpor from handling meals when the brain was compelled to higher services. Digestive, indigestive torpor is also torpor of the sense of responsibility.

In the city where I live is the point between two divisions of the Erie Railroad, each somewhat more than a hundred miles long. Before I began the agitation of the No-breakfast Plan all trainmen felt that filling their stomachs was the last duty before entering upon their taxing trips, and tired wives would have to get up at all times of the night to prepare general meals. In this city a mighty revolution for the good of wives, for the good of men themselves, and for the safety of the trains and the hapless passengers has been going on for some years.

In former times when these men came home from their rounds generally tired out, and with a feeling that in proportion to the sense of exhaustion was the need to eat, general meals had to be prepared at any time of night. All this is changed in a large measure. Trainmen have been finding out that the less food in their stomachs they take into bed with them and on to their trains, the better it is for them in every way.

More and more they are getting into the way of having a general meal when they can eat it with leisure and leisurely digest it; and I predict that a time will come when all who are in any way responsible for the running of trains will have to know how to take care of their stomachs, in order that they shall attain and maintain the highest efficiency for services where human lives so much depend on the best there is in memory, reason, and judgment. This will be a part of their preparatory education.

The "block system" has wonderfully added to the safety of the trains, but there should be a block system added to the stomachs of the dispatchers and all whose duties are so grave as the handling of human freight. There is no division so long that it cannot be doubled with less fatigue and better mental condition if the stomach be not on duty at the same time. In this I speak with the authority that comes from the study of the experiences of trainmen during many years: with one accord they speak of their trips as taken with clearer heads and stronger muscles than when large meals were thought a necessity while on duty.

With an empty stomach it takes a very long time to get into such torpor--drowsiness--as compels the after-dinner sleep. That engineer who once told me of such sleepiness as made him nod while on duty was not suffering from either lack of sleep or overwork of his body: it was simply a case of the torpor of indigestion, and this was when there was no block system to lessen the danger of such services.

There is a great deal of imperfection in what man does for man that comes from the indifference arising from the torpor of untimely food, and far more than there is any conception in what man does against man from the destruction of power in this way.

There is now one of the Erie conductors who five years ago was losing at least half of his time from asthma; there is another who was equally disabled from sudden head symptoms that would immediately disable. These men have lost no trips since they began to run their stomachs with the same care as their trains. And there is an engineer whose trips to the physician and to the drug-store for many years were as frequent as those to his engine. There has since been a half dozen years of wiser care of his stomach, and his wife says that the change for the better in his disposition is beyond description.

These men have rendered far more service, and who cannot see that these services have been of far higher character for the company, and that they have been infinitely better husbands, fathers, and citizens?

The following case will interest trainmen: D. S., a brakeman, reached the burden of two hundred and forty-six pounds, with resulting breathlessness and other ailings that taxed all his resources to perform his duties. He was induced to cut down his daily food as the only means for relief, and to add to his strength. It took him a long time to master the fact that his strength was not kept up by food, but the gradual loss of weight with the general improvement made this more and more evident. He finally reached a time when he was able to make his round trip of one hundred and ninety-six miles without a morsel of food the while, and with much less fatigue than when there was a midnight meal from a lunch-pail. Within a year the weight has gone down to one hundred and eighty-eight pounds. To my professional eye there is beauty in the bright eyes, in the condensed, smooth face, in the body enfolded with clothes that flap in the breeze like the sails of a ship. No accident will happen to precious human freight through his brain kept free from digestive torpor while on duty.

Ever since my book has been out I have been in more or less trouble with cases that badly needed my personal care, and not few in which death was inevitable. For instance, there is a woman in Illinois who has been ailing for years, and in spite of the No-breakfast Plan has had to take to her bed with acute aversion to food. Medical art had utterly failed before she changed her dietary methods.

Her dietary views are known, and so she is held in severe censure because the sick stomach is not compelled to a futile service; and though I am informed of an enlargement in the region of the bowels that has been perceptible and tender for years, her death will be considered suicidal from starvation.

A Warrensburg, Ill., editor began his fast by throwing up his food and continued it to the end; yet because he had talked about a fast it was supposed to be a case of suicide of the stupid kind; and though the post-mortem revealed a diseased gall-bladder, the doctors who made it did nothing to lessen the suicidal impression, and the death from "starvation" appeared under large headlines in the public prints.

When men as learned, able, and eminent as Dr. Shrady, of New York, go into print to inform the public that people may starve to death in ten days, and when such men as Prof. Wood, of the University of Pennsylvania, do not see any starvation in the wasting pounds of acute disease, the care of acute sickness as Nature would have it is a grave matter for the physician.

In five fatal cases under my care in which there was no possibility of feeding, there was such agitation over the question of starvation as would have subjected me to violence had my city been nearer the equator. In all these cases I was compelled to have a post-mortem to silence heathen raging. In one case in which a young man had died after weeks of inability to take food, even one of my medical brethren carried the conviction with him for years, and without seeking to inform himself, that there was a death from starvation. In this case there were spells of hunger in a fury, when meals would be taken, only to be soon thrown up, and he finally took to his bed to starve slowly to death. There was mind enough left to make a will, though the body had lost apparently more than half the normal weight; the post-mortem revealed a stomach seared, thickened, and not more than a third of the normal size.

The physiology of fasting in time of sickness is so entirely new to the medical world that every death that occurs with those who practise it is certain to be attributed to starving.

Early in this year (1900) a woman of seventy, in high circles, died from an obscure stomach trouble. For thirty-eight days there averaged nearly a half-dozen spells of vomiting; and yet it was generally believed that it was clearly a case of death from starvation, believed by those whose power to receive impressions is far stronger than their power to consider.

Fasting, because it is Nature's plan, will win the victory in all cases in which victory is possible; and yet wherever it is adopted, to become known about, there will be the same confusion of tongues as would be were violent hands laid upon gods of wood and stone in heathen temples. "Starved to death" is the verdict.

Fasting during sickness, because of the vast utility and from the impetus arising from the cases in Philadelphia, is bound to spread as by contagion; but when death occurs, all friends involved will be charged as abettors of homicide. To be fair to the opposition, and to let all readers know what chances for public censure will be theirs, whenever they see fit to let their friends recover on Nature's plan or die natural deaths, the following case is given. I quote from the Philadelphia Press of May 7, 1900:

"In the death notices of April 26 appeared the name of Mrs. Hermina Meyer, fifty years of age, of 1233 North Howard Street. At the time this short and simple record of the passing away of an ordinary, obscure woman attracted no more attention than the hundred similar names that constituted the necrological annals of April 25. But there is a startling aftermath that at once gives significance to this brief record, and rude and bitter awakening to the followers of the so-called 'Starvation Cult,' that has gained a considerable acceptance in the northeast section of the city.

"Mrs. Meyer was a believer in the fasting treatment. She was apparently a victim of this strange and heretical therapeutical faith. Kensington is buzzing with gossip concerning the deplorable death of the unfortunate woman. C. F. Meyer, the husband of the victim, accepts the death of his wife as due to heart-failure, and apparently is not disposed to complain.

"Mr. Meyer talked freely with a Press reporter yesterday concerning the sickness and death of his wife. He said that Mrs. Meyer had been ill for about a year, her malady having been diagnosed as chronic rheumatism. She had been treated by the family physician for this disease, but without relief. In despair she turned to the fasting treatment.

"From time to time she had read of the remarkable cures claimed to have been effected by complete abstention from food. Through a friend she met and talked with the family of Leonard Thress, of 2618 Frankford Avenue, whose case is proclaimed as one of the most remarkable that had been successfully treated by the fasting system. Thress was widely advertised as a victim of dropsy, who, after a complete fast of more than a month, was restored to sound health.

"Mrs. Meyer believed, and sent for Henry Ritter, the chief advocate and adviser of the fasting cult in Philadelphia. His belief in the weird treatment of disease he has adopted is seemingly unshakable.

"Ritter has superintended many cases of starvation treatment, wherein, according to his own statements, the patients have totally abstained from actual food for periods of from four to six weeks. He claims that in every case the afflicted person has completely recovered health--with the single exception of Mrs. Meyer.

"In response to her request, Ritter called upon Mrs. Meyer. She at once began her fast. Nothing was allowed to pass her lips but a small quantity of tonicum and some physiological salts, dissolved in water. Of each of these she was permitted to take sparingly every day. It is claimed by Ritter, a fact well-known to physiologists, that there is no actual food in either of these thin condiments. They are simply stimulants. These liquids, according to Ritter, are the only things given to any of the patients whose cases he has supervised.

"For twenty-five days, so says Mr. Meyer, his wife fasted and improved. At the expiration of that time, he says, her health was very much improved. She was able to walk about her room, a thing she had not been able to do for many weeks. Then there was a sudden and violent change for the worse. The patient was seized with convulsive vomiting.

"For sixteen days she suffered the excruciating pains of these convulsions. But, under Ritter's advice, Mrs. Meyer continued her fast. Till the thirty-fifth day she tasted no food. The vomiting continued unabated. On the thirty-sixth day she felt a craving for food for the first time since her long fast began. She was given oatmeal porridge. But the vomiting continued unabated.

"She grew weaker and weaker. From one hundred and fifty pounds weight she was reduced to a gaunt skeleton. When, upon the resumption of a food diet, the vomiting did not cease, the family was alarmed. The family physician was sent for in dismay. But he could do nothing. Flesh-building foods were prescribed, but they accomplished nothing. The vomiting continued, and three weeks following the breaking of the fast Mrs. Meyer died.

"The death was put down to a depleted blood-supply, or heart-failure. Ritter claimed that this unexpected turn could not have been anticipated, as the fact that the patient was subject to heart disease was previously unknown.

"He had treated her for rheumatism, and the cure was apparently in sight when heart-failure carried the patient to her grave.

"These facts were detailed by Mr. Meyer. He added that Mr. Ritter was not a physician; that he charged no fees; that he did not claim to prescribe remedies, but only advised.

"So ends the case of Mrs. Hermina Meyers, first victim of the starvation cult."

The following is from the Press of May 8:

"The death of Mrs. Hermina Meyer, after undergoing the fasting treatment for thirty-five days, has not at all shaken the faith of the adviser responsible for the ordeal, Henry Ritter, who claims to have restored tireless persons to health. He affirmed that the ravages of chronic disease had progressed too far for his treatment to conquer them, and that his attendance was advised by the family physician.

"Against this comforting declaration, however, stands the fact that the certificate of death, signed by Dr. James Chestnut, Jr., gave as the cause prolonged abstinence from food; in other words, starvation. Dr. Chestnut also has stated that the case was taken out of his hands, and Ritter installed as medical adviser, by what was virtually a dismissal. Dr. Chestnut was summoned again when the condition of the woman became critical, after twenty-five days of fasting, but she became rapidly weaker with violent convulsions and vomiting, and was beyond medical aid.

"She had never been treated for cancer of the stomach, which Ritter says he thinks she may have had, although she had a valvular affection of the heart which had existed for some time. But the fact that the cause of her death was officially attested by the family physician as due to her long fast contradicts flatly the position taken by the self-constituted healer, who made the following statement last night:

"'I have seen all the members of Mrs. Meyer's family to-day, and they are entirely satisfied that my treatment was in no way responsible for her death. I was called in at their urgent request, as their own relatives were numbered among the cures to the credit of the fasting treatment, as well as Mr. Thress. I accept no money for my work; they knew it was a labor of love, and the family physician, Dr. Chestnut, agreed with them as to the advisability of this system which they had seen tested.

"'Mrs. Meyer improved rapidly for a time, her chronic rheumatism causing her less trouble than in years, after the first three weeks of fasting. She had been treated previously for catarrh of the stomach, and it is probable that a cancer afflicted her. I am using no new system. The method has been used with very notable success by Dr. Edward H. Dewey, of Meadville, whose reputation and standing are distinguished. This is the first case I have lost out of twelve patients who had been given up as hopeless by regular physicians. It is Nature's cure, nothing more; but it was applied too late in the case of Mrs. Meyer.'

"Dr. Chestnut would not allow himself to be quoted because of the rigid rules of medical ethics. It may be stated, however, in addition to what has been said, that he does not wish to be considered as having encouraged the experiment, and that the death certificate defined his view of the responsibility."

A verdict on the part of the doctor without a post-mortem.

Against the doctor is the following, from the daughter, Miss Kate Meyer. I quote from an article in the North American of May 8, 1900:

"Mrs. Hermina Meyer, devotee of an odd cult, that regards starvation as a sure cure for all bodily ills, fasted for nearly forty days because she was suffering from rheumatism.

"The rheumatism disappeared.

"But after twenty-five days of total abstinence from food she sickened. Violent nausea came to her. She died.

"Nevertheless, Miss Kate Meyer, daughter of the dead woman, says:

"'My mother did not die because she fasted. The fasting did her good. When she began it she had been ill with rheumatism for more than a year. She could hardly walk. Her left arm was powerless. She could not lift it from her side. After two weeks of fasting she was active. She could walk. The power came back to her arm. She suffered little pain. She looked well. Then came the attacks of nausea.

"'But Dr. Chestnut, who is our family physician, was attending mother all the time. He called once a week. He said himself that the fast cure seemed to be doing mother good. When she got nausea he did not lay it to her fasting. He said it was heart trouble. That's what mother died of. Dr. Chestnut said so.

"'Do you remember the case of Leonard Thress? He cured himself of dropsy by fasting. Mother heard of it. She was introduced to Mr. Thress. He told her that all he knew of the fast cure he had learned from Henry Ritter. Mother sent and asked Mr. Ritter about the cure. Then she began it. Mr. Ritter never charged mother for anything. Dr. Chestnut consented that mother should try the Ritter cure.'

"Mrs. Meyer was the wife of Charles F. Meyer, of 1233 North Howard Street. Meyer, like his daughter, has only friendliness for Ritter, and also favors the fast cure. Mrs. Meyer, past middle age, had been sorely tried by her ailment. For more than a year Dr. Chestnut attended her, but her condition did not improve. Prescription after prescription was tested, only to fail.

"'There is little hope for me,' said the woman to her daughter. 'I'm tired of taking medicines. They do me no good.'

"She became more melancholy as the days passed. She regarded her case as hopeless. Dr. Chestnut acknowledged defeat. He had only a change of climate--a long stay in Colorado--to recommend. A very domestic woman was Mrs. Meyer. She looked with horror upon a journey. She said she would remain at home and die.

"But one day last March there gathered at a banquet in the home of Leonard Thress about a dozen persons, very happy, very healthy (or believing themselves to be so), all members of the 'starvation cure' cult.

"Each had to tell the story of a long fast that brought a remarkable cure. Newspapers gave publicity to the dinner of the little band with the odd faith in fasting. Mrs. Meyer heard of it. Here was a chance--a gleam of hope! She came to know Leonard Thress, and, through him, Henry Ritter, the apostle of the fast cure. He told her of remarkable recoveries. She caught his enthusiasm.

"But, according to Mr. Meyer, the young man was careful first that the family physician should consent. He never hinted at compensation for his services; never got it. Aside from advising total abstinence from food, he supplied small quantities of tonicum and salts dissolved in water. These contained no food matter; they were merely stimulative.

"In two weeks hope was strong with Mrs. Meyer; with all the family. Certainly, she was improving. She could walk; her arm that had been stiff and painful moved with ease--hurt no more. She still suffered occasional twinges, and decided to continue her self-imposed starvation until every rheumatic germ in her body was eradicated.

"She regarded herself as almost cured, when, after twenty-five days, she was attacked with nausea. She was very ill. It lasted sixteen days. After the first few days of fasting all desire for food had vanished. But on the thirty-sixth day she was hungry.

"Oatmeal porridge was given her sparingly. The nausea, however, did not cease. She began to grow alarmingly emaciated. She had weighed one hundred and fifty pounds. Her weight had fallen to one hundred.

"The family physician prescribed light food, but her stomach repulsed it. She grew very weak.

"On April 26 she died. Dr. Chestnut unhesitatingly issued a death certificate, ascribing her death to heart-failure. He also suspected a cancer of the stomach, but was not sure.

"Mrs. Herman Reinhardt, a cousin of the deceased woman, is firmly convinced that fasting had nothing to do with her death.

"'For more than fifteen years Mrs. Meyer suffered from some acute stomach trouble,' Mrs. Reinhardt said yesterday, 'and it is my belief that it caused her death. Her general health had been greatly benefited by abstaining from all food, but the disorder from which she suffered most could not be cured. My husband fasted for twenty-five days and was completely cured of stomach trouble, and there were no ill effects in his case.'"

The impression of this death and of these fasts upon the minds of the medical profession was perhaps fairly summed up by the eminent Horatio C. Wood, M. D., LL. D., Clinical Professor of Nervous Diseases in the University of Pennsylvania. He disregarded the legal phase of the question, the question of the legality of a layman dealing out words of cheer and comfort in cases in which the medical profession had retired in total defeat. The question had been seriously raised as to whether Mr. Ritter had not committed a crime against the laws of Pennsylvania, and for what? For simply advising these people to stop all eating until there would come a natural desire for food!

Professor Wood thus gave utterance in the Press of May 10:

"'These people are falsifying,' he said, 'There have been liars, you know, and they are not all dead. I don't believe for an instant such stories as fasting totally for forty or fifty days and keeping up energy and activity. It is contrary to common sense as well as to all we know about the human body. I don't know the object of deception, but somebody must be making money out of it, or having a craving for notoriety. It is preposterous. I understand that one of these fasters walked ten miles a day, after doing altogether without nourishment for a month or so. If these persons did what they claim to have undergone, more than one death would have been charged against the treatment, you may be sure.

"'You will remember that the professional forty-day fasters, Tanner and Suci, were reduced to mere skin and bone, were almost helpless, carefully husbanded every bit of their vital energy, and took no exercise. They were watched and studied scientifically. And here is a woman, weighing only one hundred pounds when she started fasting, claims she began to eat after thirty-eight days of starvation, and had more energy and took more exercise than in years. It is all amazingly absurd, whatever the motive may be.'"

Tanner and Suci, "skin and bones?" Cowen weighed one hundred and seventy-five pounds when he began his forty-two day fast, and lost only thirty pounds. My case of acute rheumatism revealed a loss of only forty pounds after a forty-six days' fast; and the woman of fifty-seven who began eating on the forty-third day was so well padded with muscle and fat as not to reveal the slightest suggestion of starvation as she sat down to the first meal. "Skin and bones?" This is a matter for months, and not for days.

"Falsifiers, these fasters?" Science settles important questions by investigation, not by epithet.

XVI.

As I write the closing pages of this book, the most taxing case of fasting that ever came under my care has ended in hunger, and I insert it that all may know what tribulations will be theirs if they have any part in letting their sick get well or die in that peace God and Nature clearly design for all.

A man of large mould came to me, unknown, unbidden, from a distant city on the seventeenth day of his fast. His appetite had been abolished by a severe throat and bronchial attack, both of which had been relieved before reaching me. Well posted in the theory of fasting, he came with the declared intention of fasting until hunger or death would come.

For two or three weeks he was able to be about the city with his nearly two hundred pounds of flesh; but there was an unknown, unknowable disease of the bowels and stomach in slow development. There were a dryness of the mouth and such aversion to food as to forbid all eating, and he was deaf to my suggestion that he should at least taste some of the liquid foods from time to time, to save me in the eyes of his friends from a verdict of homicide, were we to fail to win a victory. After more than fifty days without even a taste of food nausea and vomiting were added to his woes, and when his friends became aware of the many days without food no words I could utter saved me from the severest condemnation. The anxiety that involved the sick bed only depressed the patient, and when another physician had to be called to relieve the pressure the last hope with him nearly departed.

The adviser was a man of high character and of unusual general and professional acquirements. Behind him was the entire medical profession and all its literature: behind me were only Nature, many-voiced--and the patient. With us there was no lack of mutual respect, except in matters of faith and practice; but he no more tolerated my "crankiness," lunacy--perhaps imbecility--in withholding food from the sick than I his paganism in enforcing it. For the sake of the agony of friends my noble patient accepted one severe dose of medicine and one ration of predigested food. The instant response of the digestive powers was, "We have stopped business down here for repairs: when we are ready we will let you know."

Next a ration of food was sent into the sick bowels, only to cause hours of pain. The enemy having been expelled with disaster from all points of attack, there simply had to be a waiting on Nature, and in one day after the last vomiting spell there was a natural call for food--and this on the sixtieth day of the fast!

Had this man died--such was his prominence--I should have been paraded as a criminal of the stupid kind in the entire press of America, except in the papers of my own city. For this man of sixty-five, who with marvellous faith in Nature patiently waited upon her time, there promises to be many years of the days of his youth restored to him. As for me, with authorized medicine driven from the field, I see only new life unfolding in him daily, and my reward is exceeding.

Men and brethren of the medical profession: This man read his favorite Sun during every one of those sixty long days, and not one day was there revealed a hint of mental loss in clearness of apprehension. He lived because he knew that starving to death was his remotest danger; he lived also because he was made to see evidences that a cure was evolving in many ways. There was at no time apprehension, except when he felt unable to resist his friends with a No in thunder tones when it was proposed to torture him with drugs and foods.

Brethren, are you going into print to denounce the physiology or the practicality of this old method in Nature, this new method in humanity, to the sick and afflicted? Not one of you can advance arguments that will convince those who reason.

To what good end are you now enforcing your predigested foods? Are they relished better than other foods? Can they be taken with less aversion in cases of nausea and vomiting? Do they really nourish the brain so as to add clearness and strength to the mind? Do they ever prevent the uncovering of bones that makes the ways of acute sickness? If food actually can be so digested out of the body as to be ready for instant absorption, we should be able to abolish our kitchens, and at once enter upon that golden age in which there would be no dyspepsia hydraheaded; no disease of any kind, not even drunkenness, and where death would be only as the last flicker of the burned-up candle.

In this case, as in all other cases, the desire for water was abolished before hunger became marked. In this connection I will suggest to the reader that thirst is a morbid condition to be avoided as far as possible; that water is its only need, and no mortal ever needs a drop for health's sake except when thirsty. Making water-tanks of human stomachs is without the shade of physiological reason, and the alleged results for good are not based on a shade of scientific evidence: these are based wholly in the minds of the credulous enthusiasts who prescribe them. Taking large quantities of water without thirst only entails added work upon the kidneys, and thus it becomes a factor in the development of Bright's disease and other forms where the tendency exists. The actual need of water is always made clear in every case; the need always disappears before hunger can become possible.

As to the use of water on the body, this physiology has to be taken into account. The skin is covered with scales that are constantly dropping off as they mature, each to uncover a bright, clean one. As the skin is not an absorbent membrane, and as old scales are constantly dropping off, the need of frequent baths is more a need to satisfy the personal sense of cleanliness than a physiological need. These scales should not be either soaked off or brushed off in a wholesale way; the oil in the skin is a protection against weather-changes, and is also a necessity to its functional integrity, and therefore should not be dissolved and washed off by soaps that are strongly alkaline.

The body itself is very sensitive to contact with water below the natural temperature of the skin. The plunge bath is specially depressing to every human energy, and should never be indulged by the debilitated. The daily bathings of nursing children are cruel and life-depressing. Their little bodies are always clean in the physiological sense when their clothes are kept clean; hence once a week ought to satisfy all mothers.

The question of how often to bathe must be considered along these physiological lines. They whose employments soil their clothes and bodies spend the least time in cleansing their bodies; and yet in no medical work that treats of diseases and their causes is there to be found a hint that any special disease has its origin in uncleansed skin as a chronic condition. That will be a small-minded reader who draws conclusions from these statements that the author is not highly in favor of having bodies and clothes kept so habitually clean as not to be an offence to the finest fibred olfactory nerve at close range. In the use, then, of water on the body be physiologically sensible, and not the slaves of the bath-tub or "medicated" waters.

Lay readers, I draw my message to a close. I have addressed it to you because your minds are open and free. Draw near and listen while I talk rather than write. Let me look into your eyes, see the play on all the lines of expression, as I would were you in my consulting-room. Mine has reached your ears as a lone voice from the depths of some wilderness; I have tried so to speak with my pen that you could catch an echo as if from between the lines of every page.

You will not banish your medical adviser, for you still need his knowledge of the workings of disease, if you do not need the drugs you formerly believed necessary; but you will now be able in a more intelligent way to diminish the possibilities of the future need of him.

Since these wonderful fasts in Philadelphia others are occurring over the country from the contagion of example. Many are certain to be undertaken as a last resort where hope has departed; and death will come; and then there will be the confusion of tongues, as in the case of Mrs. Meyer. Her case has been the third one that I know of where the press has spread the news of death from starvation.

I have given you the case of Mrs. Meyer that you may know that no matter how hopeless any case may be considered, no matter how given up by venders of drugs, if a fast be advised and death come, death from starvation will be the general verdict. Hence on as fasts multiply, so will the press continue to make special note of all who chance to die because they had ceased to add distress to their bodies by foods that were only taken as the medicinal dose. All this you need to take into account in those cases you would advise where the medical faculty has retired in defeat.

Never in my entire professional life have I been so depressed by discordant voices as during this sixty-day fast just ended. All the air has been charged, darkened with frownings--even threats of what would happen in case of death; and as never before has this question come to me, "Why do the heathen rage and the people imagine vain things?"

Again I must tell you that the No-breakfast Plan, the plan not to eat in time of health until there are a normal need and desire for food, that are only developed after several hours of morning labor, and not to eat at all during acute sickness, is the easiest of all means to maintain health, and to regain it when lost. In my message I have had the greatest good for the greatest number of the world's busy people, who have no time to indulge abnormal, artificial ways in the recovery and maintenance of health--ways that are a real tax on time and taxing in the means involved. Passing few are they of the world's workers who have the time for all this, and especially they who are the slaves of the kitchen.

Again I must suggest to you that the actual need of daily food as a matter to meet the actual daily need is a new question in practical physiology. It may be very much less than is supposed, a matter to be determined by the scales. There are none who can eat at all with relish who are not more governed by relish than the hunger sense, as to the amount of food eaten. The real amount of daily food needed may be so small that enough of nourishment can be extracted from almost any of the easiest available foods, the main question being one of slow eating, restful eating, and with the most thorough mastication. For those who have the leisure and tastes for study over what to eat there are the works of Haig, Hoy, Hensel, Sir Henry Thompson, and others, that may be read with both interest and profit.

And now I address my last words to the mothers of the land. For you the No-breakfast Plan means the highest possible health, the greatest possible relief from the slavery of toil. On no other plan are there such promises of relief and prevention of all your sex ailings. On this plan only can you become man's equal in the hours of leisure that are his by a feeling of divine right; you also should consider the possibilities of a day of eight or ten hours as needing the reduction all the more because of your weaker bodies.

The No-breakfast Plan means for your children the best possibilities for the conservation of all the higher instincts and powers that will tend to save them from the saloon, the prison, the electric chair. If the Garden of Eden was abolished because you enticed man to eat the wrong food, it is for you to restore a new race of Adams in all the ways of health, of such health as will make the entire earth a "Paradise regained."

Readers, lay and professional, let me reiterate in my parting words, words at white heat with conviction as to their soundness and utility. Enforced food is a danger always to be measured by the gravity of the local or general disease; a danger always to be measured also by the feebleness of old age--by feebleness no matter how caused.

This physiological righteousness will remain unquestioned, its practicality unsurpassed, while man remains on the earth to violate the laws of his Creator manifest in his own body. The penalties of disobedience are as certain as that every cause is followed by a definite effect. There are no remissions in the various antitoxins; there is no hope for you through hollow needles. Nature is exacting, but she is merciful. Obey her laws that your ways may be toward Paradise, and not away from it.

###